Master   betes

The Simple, Low-Cost, Method To Normalize Blood Sugars

Keith R. Runyan MD

Master Type 1 Diabetes

Legal Notice

Copyright © 2020 by Keith R. Runyan, MD
All rights reserved.
ISBN 979-8-655976-91-7

No part of this publication may be reproduced, distributed, or transmitted in any form or by any means, including photocopying, recording, or other electronic or mechanical methods, without the prior written permission of the publisher, except in the case of brief quotations embodied in critical reviews and certain other noncommercial uses with proper citation as permitted by copyright law.

Disclaimer Notice

The information contained within this document is for educational purposes only. Every attempt has been made to provide accurate, up-to-date, reliable, and complete information. No warranties of any kind are expressed or implied. Readers acknowledge that the author is not engaging you in a doctor-patient relationship or in the rendering of legal, financial, medical, or professional advice. Consult a licensed professional before attempting any techniques outlined in this book. The author does not assume any liability or responsibility for any injuries or death related to utilizing any of the information in this book. I declare I have not received any financial support from any companies that makes products mentioned in this book. Any statements regarding insulin, medications, or products mentioned in this book are based solely on either my direct experience with them or research of them in the medical literature.

Master Type 1 Diabetes

Description

Master Type 1 Diabetes is a must read to get off the blood sugar rollercoaster and enjoy a healthy life. Written by Keith R. Runyan, MD, an internal medicine physician and nephrologist who has had type 1 diabetes since 1998, Master *Type 1 Diabetes*, describes a simple, low-cost, method to normalize blood sugars; the only effective way to prevent or reverse diabetic complications and make low blood sugars rare events. Dr. Runyan discovered his method by applying knowledge from the medical literature and self-experimentation and explains step-by-step how you can accomplish your blood sugar goals. Achieving normal blood sugars with type 1 diabetes is truly life-changing. Imagine the relief of not having to worry about the next embarrassing, unpleasant, and life-threatening low blood sugar. Image not having to worry about going blind, having your leg amputated, starting on dialysis, or dying at a young age from heart disease, all of which can occur with poorly-controlled diabetes. In short, *Master Type 1 Diabetes*, has the information you need to change your life for the better and will pay for itself hundreds of times over in the cost-savings that result from reduced insulin doses and medical expenses. Dr. Runyan posts his blood sugar results on his blog at https://ketogenicdiabeticathlete.wordpress.com/.

Table of Contents

1 – Introduction	10
Overview of the Book Contents: Chapter by Chapter	10
My Path to Normal Blood Sugars	14
Normalize Blood Sugars and Save Money Doing It	16
2 – Dr. Runyan's Life with Type 1 Diabetes	18
My Diagnosis of Type 1 Diabetes	18
Genetic and Potential Environmental Causes of Type 1 Diabetes	22
Origin of the Low-Fat High-Carbohydrate Diet	24
Beginning an Exercise Program	27
The Connection Between Diet and Disease	28
Beginning the Very Low-Carbohydrate Diet	31
Can Lifestyle Consistency Result in Normal Blood Sugars?	35
Blood Sugars in Healthy Humans	36
Finally Achieving Normal Blood Sugars	40
3 – Erratic Blood Sugars in Type 1 Diabetes	43
The Bleak State of Glycemic Control in Type 1 Diabetes	43
Why a LFHCD Causes Erratic Blood Sugars	45
Insulin, Amylin, and Glucagon Keep Blood Sugars Normal	50
Injected Insulin is Not Equivalent to β-Cell Insulin	51
Exercise Influences the Response to Exogenous Insulin	54
Insulin-on-Board	54
Muscle Insulin Sensitivity	55

Type, Duration, and Intensity of Exercise	56
Other Factors That Cause Erratic Blood Sugars	57

4 – The Low-Carbohydrate Diet — 58

Origin of the Low-Fat and Low-Carbohydrate Diets	59
Who Should Not Use a Low-Carbohydrate Diet	63
The Low-Carbohydrate Diet for Type 1 Diabetes	64
A Well-Formulated Low-Carbohydrate Diet	66
The Low-Carbohydrate Diet	69
The Very Low-Carbohydrate Diet	70
The Ketogenic Ratio	71
How to Design and Begin Your Low-Carbohydrate Diet	72
Formulating Meals with cronometer.com and dietdoctor.com	77
Why Micronutrients Matter	79
Select Your Dietary Carbohydrate Intake	81
Starch and Sugars Hidden in Processed Foods	81
Calculate Goal Bodyweight and Daily Caloric Requirement	84
Calculate Daily Dietary Protein and Fat Intake	85
How Many Meals Per Day?	88
Adjusting Dietary Fat Intake to Lose Body Fat	90
Meal Design, Timing & Muscle Protein Synthesis	91
Types of Dietary Fat in a Low-Carbohydrate Diet	92
Essential and Conditionally Essential Fatty Acids	94
Why Avoiding Vegetable Oils May Improve Health	95
Following a Low-Carbohydrate Diet While Traveling	96
The Low-Carbohydrate Diet for Vegans and Vegetarians	98

The Low-Carbohydrate Diet for Carnivores	99
Adding More Flexibility to Meals	100
Sample Day of Eating a Very Low-Carbohydrate Diet	101
Keto Chocolate Mousse Recipe	103

5 – Insulin Preparations, Dosing & Delivery — 105

Intensive Insulin Therapy	106
Exogenous Insulin Preparations for Type 1 Diabetes	108
Use of Rapid-Acting and Short-Acting Bolus Insulin	110
Use of Intermediate-Acting NPH Insulin	111
Use of Long-Acting Basal Insulin Analogs	111
Variability in Insulin Action	112
Diabetic Gastroparesis	115
Insulin-Stacking	116
Insulin Pens	119
Insulin Syringes	119
Injecting Insulin	120
Care of Insulin Vials and Pens	121
Dosing Basal Insulin	121
Dosing Bolus Insulin	123
Correction Bolus Insulin	125
Diluting Bolus Insulin	125
Adjusting Bolus Insulin with Lifestyle Changes	127
Insulin Dosing in Children and Adolescents	128
Mathematical Estimation of Bolus Insulin Doses	128
Insulin Pumps	134

The Artificial Pancreas	136

6 – Tests and Devices to Measure Glucose — 140

Hemoglobin A1c	140
Fructosamine and Glycated Albumin	143
Home Blood Glucose Meters	144
Using a Glucose Meter to Normalize Blood Sugars	145
Continuous Glucose Monitors	146

7 – Formulating an Exercise Regimen — 151

Exercise for Health and Longevity	151
Aerobic Exercise	156
Resistance Exercise	157
High Intensity Interval Training	158
Exercise Training Improves Insulin Sensitivity	159
Insulin-on-Board and the Blood Sugar Response to Exercise	160
Varying Insulin Sensitivity Adversely Affects Blood Sugars	161
Intense Exercise Can Release Counterregulatory Hormones	163
Consistent Daily Exercise to Achieve Normal Blood Sugars	164
How to Structure Your Exercise Plan	166
Compensating for Exercise in Children	168
Avoiding Exercise-Related Hypoglycemia	168

8 – Sleep, Sunshine, Alcohol & Tobacco — 170

Sleep, Sunshine, and Circadian Rhythms	170
Alcohol Use In Those With Diabetes	172
Tobacco Use In Those With Diabetes	174

9 – Medications & Hormones Affecting Blood Sugars — 175
Medications — 175
SGLT2 Inhibitors — 177
Stress Hormones — 178
Hormonal Changes During Menstrual Cycles — 179

10 – Hypoglycemia — 181
Hypoglycemia in Type 1 Diabetes — 181
Physiologic Response to Hypoglycemia — 184
Symptomatic Response to Hypoglycemia — 185
The Dangers of Hypoglycemia & Hypoglycemia Unawareness — 186
Treatment of Hypoglycemia — 188
Prevention of Hypoglycemia — 190

11 – Lipoproteins, CVD, Metformin & Symlin — 193
Low-Carbohydrate Diets & Elevations of LDL-C — 193
Reducing Cardiovascular Disease Risk in Those With T1D — 197
Is There Evidence That a LCD Prevents CVD? — 198
Metformin — 199
Pramlintide (Symlin) — 203

12 – Improving Body Composition — 205
Extent and Causes of Excess Body Fat in T1D — 205
The Consequences of Excess Body Fat in T1D — 208
Losing Body Fat While Achieving Normal Blood Sugars — 210
Physical Activity Facilitates Body Fat Loss — 214
Compliance & Consistency — 215

Obesity Medicine Physician Consultation	217

13 – Ketosis & Diabetic Ketoacidosis — 219

Ketones and Nutritional Ketosis	219
Measuring Ketones When Following a VLCD	221
Diabetic Ketoacidosis	223
Medium-Chain Triglycerides, Coconut Oil, and MCT Oil	225
Known and Potential Benefits of Nutritional Ketosis	226

14 – Low-Carb Diet Myths — 228

Myth 1: A High-Protein LCD Can Injure Healthy Kidneys	228
Myth 2: A High-Protein VLCD is Not Ketogenic	229
Myth 3: Dietary Carbohydrates Are Needed For Brain Energy	233
Myth 4: Low-Carbohydrate Diets Are Nutrient Deficient	235
Myth 5: Low-Carbohydrate Diets Cause Osteoporosis	235
Myth 6: Low-Carbohydrate Diets Cause Muscle Wasting	236
Myth 7: Low-Carbohydrate Whole Foods Are Expensive	238
Myth 8: Glargine (Lantus) Insulin Increases Cancer Risk	239
Diabetes And Weight-Management Coaching	240
Comments, Book Reviews, Suggestions, Are All Welcome	240

Table of Abbreviations — 242

Table of References — 245

1 – Introduction

"It always seems impossible until it is done."
Nelson Mandela, anti-apartheid leader, and former President of South Africa.

"Our greatest glory is not in never falling, but in rising every time we fall."
Confucius, Chinese philosopher.

Overview of the Book Contents: Chapter by Chapter

I wish I could have read this book in 1998 when I was diagnosed with type 1 diabetes mellitus (T1D). I offer it to you in the hopes you can use it to normalize your blood sugars and restore your potential for a healthy life without the constant threat of low blood sugars (hypoglycemia) and diabetic complications. As a physician, I have known for a long time that being healthy is our most valuable asset, but developing T1D myself put that axiom into sharper focus. This book presents new diabetes management skills and lifestyle habits specifically tailored to help those with T1D to normalize blood sugars, lose body fat, dramatically reduce the frequency of hypoglycemia, and as a result, feel energetic and enjoy life! I hope I can inspire everyone to adopt them because the benefits are immeasurable. The diabetes management skills and lifestyle habits I present do not need to adopted overnight, but rather can be added over time at your own pace. I certainly discovered and implemented them myself over many years. Diabetes management skills that contribute to normalization of blood sugars include frequent blood glucose monitoring by blood glucose meter or continuous glucose monitor (CGM), consistent timing and quantification of meals, exercise, and insulin administration, and proper selection of insulin administered via injections or pump to match your unique physiology. Lifestyle habits that contribute to normalization of blood sugars include consistent low-carbohydrate, whole-food, nutrient-dense meals, consistent daily exercise, and prudent sleep hygiene, all of which result in reduced and predictable insulin doses. This book focuses on these unique strategies and is not intended to be a comprehensive text on the management of all aspects of T1D. I did not set out to discover a low-cost method to normalize blood sugars, it just turns out that 1) whole foods can be less expensive than processed foods, 2) taking less insulin is less expensive, 3) being healthy reduces medical expenses, and 4) since my method does not require an insulin pump or CGM, normal blood sugars can be achieved without incurring the cost of purchasing these devices and their ongoing supplies. That said, use of an insulin pump or CGM is perfectly compatible with my method and, honestly, using a CGM has advantages for many with T1D. It was developed over a 12-year period beginning with a program of regular exercise, then adopting a low-carbohydrate dietary lifestyle, and later adding quantification, consistency and timing of meals, insulin injections, exercise, and sleep habits to normalize my blood sugars. Today, I can say that my blood sugar control is that of a nondiabetic person. I have reversed my diabetic complications, I take half as much insulin (at half the cost), I feel energetic, and most importantly, I no longer worry about having hypoglycemic episodes because they are so mild and infrequent. This book describes exactly what I did and how you can adopt some or all of the components of the program to suit your needs and preferences to improve your blood sugars, health, and longevity. A normal life with T1D is possible; all you need is the correct information, motivation, and direction to adjust your lifestyle and diabetes management skills. For your

safety, you should continue to engage with your healthcare provider while on this journey. I do offer online diabetes coaching for those who need help adapting the strategies to their particular situation at
https://ketogenicdiabeticathlete.wordpress.com/coaching/.

The book begins in Chapter 2 with my 20 plus-year journey of dealing with, and finally conquering T1D, using the simple, low-cost method I developed. Chapter 3 reviews the many causes of erratic blood sugars experienced by those with T1D. It is helpful to understand these causes since minimizing or eliminating them is a key aspect of my method. Because all forms of diabetes including T1D are characterized by marked dietary carbohydrate intolerance, my method starts with adopting a whole-food, nutrient-dense, low-carbohydrate diet (LCD) or very low-carbohydrate diet (VLCD) explained in detail in Chapter 4. It is important to know that a LCD is a safe dietary pattern for those with T1D. I do list some rare genetic conditions that are contraindications to using a LCD. I will teach you how to formulate your LCD to be nutritionally complete, with enough protein to build and preserve your lean muscle mass and support athletic pursuits, and with enough healthful fat to improve body composition. I discuss how to avoid the common mistakes made when implementing a LCD. Coupled with the LCD, I explain how to design a more consistent schedule of quantified meals, another important technique to normalize blood sugars. I then explain in Chapter 5 how to choose an insulin regimen administered via injections or pump and to calculate a dose estimate to match consistent meals and physical activity. The utility and pitfalls of hemoglobin A1c (HbA1c), fructosamine, glycated albumin, blood glucose meters, and CGM are discussed in Chapter 6. Chapter 7 explains why one should exercise as part of living a healthy and functional life and how to establish an exercise program that allows for normal blood sugars. I explain why intermittent physical activity can make controlling blood sugars more difficult, but that once a regular exercise regimen is established, muscle insulin sensitivity and blood sugar control stabilizes. I discuss the effect of sleep, sunshine exposure, and your body's built-in circadian clock on blood sugar regulation and how to adjust them to reduce variation in blood sugars (glycemic variation) in Chapter 8. Chapter 9 covers the topics of illness, stress hormones, sex hormones, and medications that can cause erratic blood sugars. Chapter 10 discusses the very important topic of hypoglycemia in T1D. I review the causes, symptoms, dangers, treatment, and most importantly, the prevention of hypoglycemia. In Chapter 11, I discuss the meaning of elevations in low-density lipoprotein cholesterol (LDL-C) that can occur in a minority of those adopting a LCD and dietary manipulations that may improve it. I also discuss how normalizing blood sugars reduces the risk of cardiovascular disease (CVD), the leading cause of death in those with diabetes, as well as the use of metformin and pramlintide (Symlin) in T1D to improve insulin sensitivity and further reduce insulin doses. Since about half of those with T1D are overweight [Mottalib, A, et al., 2017], I address the reasons we should improve body composition and specific measures to lose excess body fat in Chapter 12. In Chapter 13, I explore ketones — why and how we make them on a VLCD — and discuss the difference between nutritional ketosis and diabetic ketoacidosis (DKA). In Chapter 14, I discuss some common myths about the use of a LCD/VLCD for the treatment of T1D. The Table of Abbreviations defines abbreviations used in the book. The Table of References includes more than 300 medical and scientific references for those who want to deepen their knowledge of the topics covered in this book. The references are listed alphabetically by the first author's last name and year of publication. The copy and search functions can be used in the Kindle version to locate references from within the text.

My Path to Normal Blood Sugars

You may wonder why it took a physician twelve years, i.e., 2007 to 2019, to devise the method presented in this book. I assure you the delay was not due to lack of motivation, but rather due to a lack of information available at the time of my diagnosis in 1998 and for many years thereafter. Additionally, it wasn't until more recently that I even thought it might be possible for a person with T1D to have normal blood sugars. Now that I have achieved normal blood sugars, I want you to have this information so that you can accomplish it as well. I acquired this information both from extensive study of the medical literature and popular books written by other physicians, as well as numerous self-experiments. I have tried many different versions of VLCD and LCD. I tried seven different insulin preparations and scores of insulin-administration schedules and dosing combinations. I have devised dozens of exercise regimens in a wide range of types, intensities, and durations from swimming, cycling, and running to bodybuilding, powerlifting, and olympic weightlifting. I have learned how to increase and decrease my bodyweight for masters olympic weightlifting while still controlling blood sugars. I have had thousands of hypoglycemic episodes, more than I care to mention, but eventually learned how to make them infrequent events. I have measured urine, breath, and blood ketone levels and experimented with coconut oil and medium-chain triglyceride (MCT) oil to manipulate my ketone levels. The primary motivation for all of this experimentation has been to find a systematic way to first, avoid hypoglycemic episodes, and second, to normalize my blood sugars while still living a full and physically-active life. I hope you will be able to benefit from my research and self-experimentation to normalize your blood sugars in a compressed time-window. I have had many failures in my attempts, but I enthusiastically moved on from my failures without thinking that preventing hypoglycemia and achieving normal blood sugars would be impossible. I can say it has been a long path to reach my current level of success, but the results have been well worth the effort and I hope I can convince you of the same. While I feel I have the upper hand on my T1D, I know there will be occasions when my blood sugars will stray from my intended goal and that there will always be room for improvement. I will not stop trying to improve every aspect of my health since it is my most valuable asset.

The solution I have devised is not even close to what I was taught in medical school or during my post-graduate medical training in internal medicine and nephrology. While attending Emory University School of Medicine from 1982 to 1986, nutrition education was not emphasized, but had it been covered, would likely have been wrong as I will discuss later. Only more recently did I learn that many medical treatments are implemented before they are tested and found to be effective. In medicine, both science-based and untested treatments are handed down from one generation of physicians to the next as if they are of equal validity. Questioning authority and scientific dogma in medicine is discouraged and often ridiculed. Many of those who challenged the dogma were ousted from their academic positions, lost their research funding, or at best were simply ignored. This applies to the nutritional treatment of T1D and type 2 diabetes mellitus (T2D) with a low-fat high-carbohydrate diet (LFHCD). Its use, based on a hypothesis, rather than tested science, is discussed in more detail in Chapter 2.

With this perspective, I think you will have a better understanding of why your physician(s) may not have discussed nutrition with you, or if they have, that you were told something quite different than what I will be telling you in this book. Typically, your diabetes care team serves as well-meaning advisors. Your visits with them are short, occur infrequently, and focus on refilling your medications, reviewing your lab results, and referring you to specialists to address your long-term complications. But the day-to-day management of blood sugar is YOUR responsibility. By following a LFHCD as recommended, your blood sugars will be high and erratic with frequent hypoglycemia and a HbA1c of 6.5–7% at best. HbA1c is a measure of glycated-hemoglobin and, in most cases, is indicative of the average blood glucose over the previous three months (see Chapter 6). During your visit, much less attention is given to strategies to improve blood sugar control, let alone, normalize it. Since healthcare providers rarely, if ever, see a patient with T1D with normal blood sugars, they, as was I, are not aware it is even possible, nor have they learned how to normalize it. I encourage you to give your physician a copy of this book. By reading it, they will be better prepared to help you and others with T1D.

Normalize Blood Sugars and Save Money Doing It

My objective is to teach you the strategies, based on both scientific principles and anecdotal experience, that have worked for me and my online clients to achieve normal glycemia. I do not claim that my method is the one and only effective method; just that it is one effective method. I would also like to be a source of hope and inspiration to those who struggle with trying to regulate their blood sugars and avoid hypoglycemia. I feel like I can be a proof-of-concept that normal glycemia is achievable and spread the knowledge I have acquired to help others manage their T1D more effectively and safely. I hope you will be able to use my method to optimize your blood sugars and enjoy the positive results of doing so. Once armed with the proper information and a willingness to make the necessary lifestyle changes, I think the majority of those with T1D can achieve normal blood sugars with minimal high and low blood sugars and reverse all but the most advanced or end-stage diabetic complications, shed body fat, restore health and vigor, and gain the peace-of-mind that results from these improvements.

Using the strategies presented in this book, comes the additional benefit of reducing the financial costs associated with caring for diabetes including 1) lower insulin costs due to lower insulin doses, 2) lower hospital bills for emergency room visits for hypoglycemia, diabetic ketoacidosis (DKA), or treating the consequences of long-term diabetic complications, 3) whole, nutritious, LCD foods are less expensive than convenient, ready-to-eat, processed foods, fast-food, or dining out at restaurants, and 4) not needing to purchase expensive technologies and supplies including an insulin pump and CGM. While the method presented in this book will work with an insulin pump and CGM, there are many with T1D who can't afford these devices and they too need a means to achieve normal glycemia.

2 – Dr. Runyan's Life with Type 1 Diabetes

"Ever tried. Ever failed. No Matter. Try Again. Fail again. Fail better."
Samuel Beckett, author of *Worstward Ho*.

"He who has a why to live for, can bear with almost any how."
Friederick Nietzche, German philosopher.

Before I describe in detail how I normalized my blood sugars, let me introduce myself to you in more detail so that you can understand the road I traveled before writing this book. In addition to my story, I will intersperse some important concepts and background information about T1D, diet, and metabolism.

My Diagnosis of Type 1 Diabetes

I was diagnosed with T1D at the age of 38 in 1998. More specifically, I was diagnosed with a form of T1D called latent autoimmune diabetes in adults (LADA) [Stenström, G, et al., 2005]. T1D is caused by the autoimmune destruction of the beta-cells (β-cells) in the pancreas whose function is to monitor and regulate blood glucose by appropriately secreting insulin and amylin. The primary difference between LADA and T1D is that the rate of β-cell destruction is slower in LADA compared to T1D. In contrast to T1D, having LADA can lead to two difficulties: 1) being incorrectly diagnosed as T2D and treated as such, and 2) having abnormally high blood sugars for a longer period of time before the diagnosis is made. The later occurred in my case, in large part, due to denial of my illness. By contrast, if LADA is diagnosed early on, one has the opportunity to normalize blood sugars as described in this book, avoid possible environmental triggers, and perhaps slow the rate of β-cell destruction. Unfortunately, multiple clinical trials of different immune altering medications have been unable to stop the inexorable destruction of the β-cells. A large study [Rewers, M, et al., 2018] is exploring multiple possible environmental causes of T1D, but results are still pending. Treatment of LADA is essentially the same as T1D, to replace the insulin deficiency with exogenous insulin (insulin from outside the body). The amount of exogenous insulin needed to correct blood sugar is determined by the degree of one's β-cell destruction and insulin sensitivity which can vary quite significantly from person to person and in an individual as time passes. In most cases of T1D, a 'honeymoon' period follows the initial diagnosis such that insulin doses are low or can be temporarily stopped. This occurs because the initial insulin therapy resolves the high blood sugars (hyperglycemia) which suppressed the ability of the remaining functioning β-cells to secrete insulin. Over time, as β-cell destruction continues, one's exogenous insulin requirements will increase. Within months to years after the diagnosis, most of the β-cells will have been destroyed. In my case, I postponed seeing a physician and getting a diagnosis to the point that I had no honeymoon period.

My symptoms of LADA began sometime in 1996 while working as an emergency-room physician. I first started losing weight, albeit slowly. I was not in the habit of weighing myself and thus was unable to assess the rate of weight loss. Because I had no other symptoms, I was not concerned, although I should have been in retrospect. Then in 1997, I started having diarrhea, infrequently at first, then as time passed, it become more frequent. I thought it was due to a food intolerance and maybe that was why I was losing weight. I tried eliminating foods, one after another for many months, without any improvement. In 1998 as I continued losing weight, I noticed a generalized fatigue and by the summer, I was having increased urinary frequency, thirst, and hunger that never seemed satisfied. I had been in complete denial that I had a serious medical condition. In September 1998, I finally decided I had better find out the cause of my symptoms. The initial blood tests revealed my fasting blood glucose was 389 mg/dl (21.6 mmol/l or mM), easily making the diagnosis of diabetes. Note: divide mg/dl by 18 to get mM. In light of this diagnosis, the cause of my diarrhea was 'diabetic diarrhea' due to autonomic neuropathy: a complication of long-standing hyperglycemia. I drove from the physician's office to the pharmacy and immediately started on intermediate-acting insulin, NPH (Humulin N), as my basal insulin and regular human insulin (Humulin R) as my mealtime bolus insulin. These were the insulin preparations I was accustomed to prescribing during my medical training. Over the next several months, the insulin therapy allowed me to regain my lost muscle and body fat, but I also developed new symptoms related to the rapid lowering of blood sugar. I noticed blurred vision as well as fluid retention in my ankles for the next several weeks. Insulin signals the kidneys to retain both sodium and water which explained the fluid in my ankles. Another unexpected effect of my insulin therapy was the unmasking of both autonomic and peripheral neuropathy due to the rapid lowering of blood glucose. In addition to diabetic diarrhea, I developed 1) pain and numbness of the skin over my entire body from the top of my scalp to the tip of my toes (peripheral neuropathy of sensory nerves), 2) profuse sweating and heat that began soon after eating (gustatory sweating from autonomic neuropathy), 3) dry skin in my feet and lower legs (peripheral neuropathy of nerves controlling sweat and sebaceous glands), 4) dizziness on standing (orthostatic hypotension from autonomic neuropathy), 5) erectile dysfunction (autonomic neuropathy), and 6) depression (common with major illnesses). I tried ≈ 10–15 medications over a 9-month period to relieve these symptoms without any perceivable benefits. I was hopeful that if I did a very good job of managing my blood sugar, my symptoms would eventually dissipate. With time, my symptoms of neuropathy did gradually remit, but at different rates. The total body pain, gustatory sweating, erectile dysfunction, and depression took about a year to resolve. The diabetic diarrhea took about three years to resolve. The orthostatic hypotension and numbness and dryness of the skin in my legs and feet improved slowly over time, but took about 16 years to completely resolve. The lack of any improvement of my neuropathic symptoms with multiple medications and their resolution with near-normal blood sugars lead me to believe addressing the root cause is the most effective treatment for diabetic complications. I am fortunate to have never developed diabetic retinopathy (diabetic eye disease) or nephropathy (diabetic kidney disease) or any vascular disease (my coronary artery calcium score was zero on 4/24/2018 at age 57). I am also fortunate to have never had DKA or required hospitalization for diabetes.

In addition to dealing with the pain and discomfort of my autonomic and peripheral neuropathy, I encountered another problem soon after starting insulin: hypoglycemia. Hypoglycemia is defined by a blood glucose < 70 mg/dl (or 3.9 mM) often associated with a large variety of very unpleasant symptoms. It is caused by unintentional excessive exogenous insulin administration. The vast majority of those with T1D have experienced this problem. Not only is hypoglycemia unpleasant, it is also embarrassing and potentially deadly. For the first 14 years after my diagnosis, my HbA1c was usually 6.5–7%. This is the degree of blood sugar control that physicians and diabetes organizations currently recommend. Because I was eating a LFHCD, I had anywhere from two to five symptomatic hypoglycemic episodes each week which prevented me from achieving normal blood sugars. They could occur at any time, but it seemed most common after meals due to the mismatch between mealtime bolus insulin and meal macronutrients. I did have some episodes at night (nocturnal hypoglycemia) that lead me to switch my basal insulin from NPH to lente in 2000, and later, to ultralente insulin in 2002. When a basal insulin has a peak of action, it increases the likelihood of nocturnal hypoglycemia. NPH has a more pronounced peak of action than any of the basal insulin analogs on the market (lente and ultralente were discontinued). In 2003, I switched from ultralente to glargine (Lantus) as my basal insulin. Lantus further reduced my nocturnal hypoglycemia and I used it for 16 years until November 22, 2019 when I switched to degludec (Tresiba). In 2000, I switched from Humulin R to lispro (Humalog) as my mealtime bolus insulin with improvement in post-meal hyperglycemia. Because hypoglycemia is so ubiquitous in those with T1D, I will discuss it in greater detail in Chapter 10 and review all of the currently available insulin preparations in Chapter 5.

Genetic and Potential Environmental Causes of Type 1 Diabetes

In the United States, 1 in 300 (0.3%) will be diagnosed with T1D. Of all the new cases of T1D, 42% occur in those over the age of 30 years [Thomas, NJ, et al., 2018]. Of those who develop T1D, more than 85% of cases are sporadic, meaning no first degree relatives have T1D. Relatives of the person with T1D are at higher risk of developing T1D: offspring 1%, sibling 3.2–6%, dizygotic twin 6%, and monozygotic twin 50%. Genes play a role in determining one's risk of developing T1D, the major histocompatibility complex on chromosome 6 being the most important, and, in particular, the HLA class II molecules (DR, DQ, and DP). The number of new cases of T1D has increased by 1.4% annually between 2002 and 2012 [Mayer-Davis, EJ, et al., 2017] and by 1.9% annually between 2012 and 2015 [Divers, J, et al., 2020]. Such a rapid increase could not be explained by our genes alone and requires identification of lifestyle and/ or environmental causes which, so far, have remained elusive [Michels, A, et al., 2015]. Possibilities include 1) viruses: enterovirus, Coxsackie B virus, rotavirus, mumps virus, cytomegalovirus, and rubella virus [Filippi, CM, et al., 2008], 2) dietary antigens: A1 β-casein, a cow's milk protein (not present in goat, sheep, and other ruminant's milk) [Chia, JSJ, et al., 2017], and gliadin or gluten [Fasano, A, 2011, Achenbach, P, et al., 2005], 3) an abnormal microbiome [Zheng, P, et al., 2018], and 4) vitamin D deficiency in infancy [Chia, JSJ, et al., 2017]. A healthy small intestine absorbs only small molecules and excludes larger molecules, viruses, and bacteria. However, certain infectious agents or dietary substances can disrupt our intestinal permeability, opening the tight-junctions between the enterocytes lining the intestinal wall, allowing foreign substances to enter our bloodstream. These foreign substances become targets for attack by our immune system that can also mistakenly attack our own tissues in the process causing various autoimmune diseases. This review article [Fasano, A, 2011] explains that, "A fast-growing number of diseases are recognized to involve alterations in intestinal permeability related to changes in tight-junction competency. These comprise autoimmune diseases, including T1D, celiac disease, multiple sclerosis, and rheumatoid arthritis, in which intestinal tight-junctions allow the passage of antigens from the intestinal milieu, challenging the immune system to produce an immune response that can target any organ or tissue in genetically predisposed individuals. Tight-junctions are also involved in cancer development, infections, and allergies." In the case of T1D, this autoimmune process winds up targeting and destroying the β-cells in the process. This process of autoimmune attack by our immune system is initiated by the B lymphocytes (or B cells) which produce autoantibodies reactive to four autoantigens (islet cell autoantibodies or ICA): insulinoma-associated antigen-2 (I-A2, ICA512), insulin (micro IAA or mIAA), glutamic acid decarboxylase 65 (GAD65), and zinc transporter 8 (ZnT8). B cells present antigen to diabetogenic CD4 and CD8 T lymphocytes (or T cells) which infiltrate the islets of Langerhans in the pancreas resulting in β-cell destruction [Van Belle, TL, et al., 2011]. Celiac disease occurs in a larger percentage of those with T1D compared to the general population, thus linking gliadin as a potential causative agent in both of these diseases. Checking for IgA tissue transglutaminase antibodies is a laboratory test to screen for celiac disease. Some of the beneficial effects of a LCD in those with T1D might result from the complete exclusion of gliadin and gluten in grains — wheat, rye, barley, kamut, spelt, teff, and couscous — that would facilitate healing of the tight-junctions, although research is needed to confirm this hypothesis. This study [Mäkimattila, S, et al., 2020] from Finland found that 22.8% of those with T1D had at least one additional autoimmune disease, autoimmune hypothyroidism (under-active thyroid) being the most common. Thus, persons with T1D should have their thyroid function, i.e., TSH (thyroid stimulating hormone) level, checked and also consider testing for antithyroid peroxidase and antithyroglobulin antibodies per their physician's guidance. I also believe my years of sleep deprivation, from 1986 through 1998, contributed to my development of T1D. As little as one night of sleep deprivation results in both liver and muscle insulin resistance on the following day [Donga, E, et al., 2010]. I discuss the role of sleep habits on blood sugar management in Chapter 8.

Origin of the Low-Fat High-Carbohydrate Diet

After my diagnosis of T1D, when I finally found time to look for information about diet, the American Diabetes Association (ADA) was recommending the same LFHCD that I had been following my entire life. I purchased an endocrinology textbook, *Ellenberg & Rifkin's Diabetes Mellitus*, [Porte, Jr, R. et al., 1997] to learn more about managing T1D.

Chapter 30 titled, *Nutritional Management Of The Person With Diabetes,* reviewed the history of nutritional recommendations for diabetes that ranged from very-low to very-high in dietary carbohydrate, from very-low to very-high in dietary fat, and from primarily animal-foods to primarily plant-foods. The textbook pointed out that much controversy existed concerning the dietary management of diabetes. They noted that: "Between 1940 and 1970, the ADA recommended carbohydrate restriction [20% of energy from dietary carbohydrate], a view that was reversed with the 1971 revisions and reaffirmed with the 1979 and 1986 *Nutritional Recommendations and Principles for Individuals with Diabetes Mellitus*. In essence, the revised recommendations were to restrict fat, limit protein intake to the recommended daily intake (RDI), 0.8 g/kg/d of protein, and fill the void with carbohydrates. These principles were based on new information and a growing concern for the role of lipids in macrovascular disease [i.e., cardiovascular disease (CVD)] and of protein intake upon renal [kidney] integrity [see Chapter 14]. Although most of the recommendations were based on scientific information, there are clearly limitations imposed on the recommendations because of the paucity of hard data to support the recommendations that are offered on the basis of clinical experience and consensus."

While the document mentioned the limitations of its recommendations, I and many others reading it, trusted the experts' recommendations. We know now there is no evidence that a LFHCD protects against CVD [Harcombe, Z, et al., 2016]. For those with either T1D or T2D, both characterized by dietary carbohydrate intolerance, recommending a LFCHD worsens glycemic control and increases the risk of CVD [Aronson, D, et al., 2002]. There was evidence dating back to the 1950s that dietary carbohydrates, and in particular sugar, caused elevated blood triglyceride levels (hypertriglyceridemia) and was associated with CVD [Albrink, MJ, et al., 1959].

The diabetes textbook [Porte, Jr, R. et al., 1997] also stated: "Furthermore, restrictions regarding the consumption of sucrose are no longer justified based on studies that show similar effects of sucrose and starches on glycemia." Regrettably, from this I concluded that I could continue eating milk chocolate, candy, and other desserts after developing diabetes since they were equivalent to all other carbohydrates as long as I included it in my carbohydrate count. Following this advice was obviously a mistake in retrospect, but it was just one of many I have made over the years. I try not to dwell on my mistakes, but rather learn from them, and continue to improve. Only after totally eliminating sugar from my diet in 2011 did I realize I had an addiction to sugar. Because the LCD completely excludes all added sugar and minimizes natural sugars, I won't be focusing much on the harmful effects of sugar other than to list a few of the conditions it causes when consumed in sufficient quantities: 1) dental caries, 2) high blood pressure, 3) insulin resistance, 4) metabolic syndrome, 5) obesity, 6) T2D, 7) CVD, and 8) non-alcoholic fatty liver disease (NAFLD), i.e., fat deposition in the liver [Nakagawa, T, et al., 2006]. Since more than 70% of processed foods have added sugar [Ng, SW, et al., 2012], this is another reason I strongly suggest avoiding them altogether.

In 2001, I started a solo private practice in nephrology in St. Petersburg, Florida. Nephrology is a subspecialty of internal medicine that deals with high blood pressure, mineral and electrolyte disturbances, and diseases of the kidneys. Although I was no longer working night-shifts in the emergency department, I was now on-call seven nights a week from home for hospital consults and patients in my practice. Thus my sleep was interrupted most nights for the next 13 years. This likely contributed to my difficulties managing my blood sugars.

At work, hypoglycemic episodes were especially embarrassing because I felt a physician should know how to prevent them, but I couldn't. This prompted me to eliminate lunch and eat two meals/day, simply to reduce the number of hypoglycemic episodes related to taking insulin with lunch. From this experience I can say that eating two meals/day is a doable strategy for those who want to reap the potential benefits of intermittent fasting [de Cabo, R, et al., 2019].

Beginning an Exercise Program

By 2007, my private practice was well-established, so I decided I had better start doing some regular exercise to improve my health. I enjoyed sports having done gymnastics, wrestling, and cross-country running in school. I also enjoyed riding my bike growing up. In 2007, my wife had started training for and entering triathlons, so I decided to join in with her. All I had to do was learn how to swim efficiently and get back in shape. While I definitely enjoyed the physical activity, doing it with T1D was more challenging than I had anticipated. It didn't take very long to figure out that aerobic exercise commonly leads to hypoglycemia if no pre-exercise adjustments are made, i.e., taking food, glucose (dextrose), or reducing insulin doses. In the sport of triathlon, 'sports nutrition' products were touted as 'necessary' to fuel muscles during exercise. Only years later did it become clear that consuming sugar during exercise is not required once one adapts to a LCD [Volek, JS, et al., 2016]. Since I needed something to prevent hypoglycemia, I used the sports nutrition products that the other athletes were consuming. They consisted of various forms of sugar, mainly sucrose and maltodextrin (chains of dextrose made from corn), with some amino acids and caffeine in convenient packages that could be opened and consumed while cycling or running. I soon learned that the amount consumed made the difference between low, normal, or high blood sugar, but determining the right dose was indeed difficult. My tendency was to overdo it. I was fearful of developing hypoglycemia while riding my bike alone. With time, I learned how different types, intensity, and duration of exercise affected my blood sugar as well as how to adjust insulin doses and use dextrose rather than sports nutrition products during training. In 2010, I had built enough endurance to complete a half-ironman distance triathlon. This one-day event typically starts with a 1.2-mile open water swim in a lake, river, or ocean, followed by a 56-mile bike ride, and finishes with a 13.1-mile half-marathon. Since these events are too long to rehearse in advance, I was unable to practice blood sugar management strategies prior to the event. Thus, each event was my experiment. Some went well, while others, not so well. I remember in one half-ironman event, I injected 3 international units (IU) of lispro (Humalog) while riding my bike for a blood sugar in the 300s mg/dl (16s mM). I finished with a blood glucose of ≈ 150 mg/dl (≈ 8.3 mM), but it seemed to me that these high blood sugars would not be 'health-promoting' in the long-term which was the reason I started exercising in the first place.

The Connection Between Diet and Disease

In 2011, I decided that I wanted to do a full ironman-distance event. I just wanted to see if I could do it, but I knew my blood sugar management could be a potential problem given my experience so far. While training on my stationary bike one day, I heard a podcast interview with Loren Cordain, PhD. He was talking about the Paleo Diet and what struck me was his explanation about the close connection between novel changes in diet and chronic disease. If he were correct, I wondered why such a connection between these novel foods and disease was not emphasized in medical school. I had to find out if this connection was fact or fiction. I read Dr. Cordain's book, *The Paleo Diet* [Cordain, L, 2011]. One thing was clear from his book, humans only recently started eating refined and processed foods like sugar, flour, white rice, and vegetable oils that require advanced technologies to produce. The introduction of these refined foods also coincided with an increasing incidence of multiple diseases almost exclusively found in Western civilizations beginning in the 1800s. This was surprising to me given that the majority of my workday was spent treating these same novel diseases with medications.

In November 2011, I changed my diet to the Paleo diet. I eliminated all grains (wheat, corn, oats, barley, rice, etc.), refined carbohydrates, sugar, potatoes, legumes, dairy, vegetable oils, and processed foods, but added more whole fruit, along with my usual meat, fish, eggs, and an assortment of nonstarchy vegetables. I did miss eating certain foods, but never felt a strong craving to eat them. Because I had been saving all my blood sugar readings and insulin doses on log sheets since 2007, I was able to calculate that on the Paleo Diet my average or mean blood glucose was 145 mg/dl (8.1 mM) and standard deviation of blood glucose was 79 mg/dl (4.9 mM), both much higher than normal. Standard deviation of blood glucose (SDBG) is an easily calculated measure of glycemic variability (variation in blood glucose) and equals the square root of the variance, where variance is the arithmetic mean of the square of the differences between each blood glucose measurement and the mean blood glucose. By squaring the difference, the variance and SDBG put more weight, or emphasis, on the contribution of blood glucose values that are far from the mean, i.e., very-high or very-low blood glucose values. Thus for a person with T1D, a normal SDBG means that very-high and very-low blood glucose readings must be quite infrequent. Another useful statistic is the coefficient of variation (COV). This is simply the SDBG divided by the mean blood glucose, expressed as a percentage. Using the COV allows one to compare glycemic variability from different time periods when the mean blood glucose was different or when the unit of measure is different, e.g., mg/dl versus mM. My COV on the Paleo Diet was 54%. My total daily insulin dose (TDID) decreased from 52.2 IU/day to 38.2 IU/day (a 27% reduction). Although the Paleo Diet is not a LCD, per se, I was eating fewer carbohydrates having eliminated sugar, bread, potatoes, pasta, rice, and all desserts. The frequency of hypoglycemic episodes did not improve on the Paleo Diet and I continued searching for a solution. I heard interviews with Richard K. Bernstein, MD, Gary Taubes, and Stephen Phinney, MD, PhD on Jimmy Moore's podcast: *Livin La Vida Low-Carb Show*. I read their books, *Dr. Bernstein's Diabetes Solution* [Bernstein, RK, 2011], *Good Calories, Bad Calories* [Taubes, G, 2007], and *The Art and Science of Low Carbohydrate Living* [Volek, JS, et al., 2011a] and *The Art and Science of Low Carbohydrate Performance* [Volek, JS, et al., 2011b]. I consider these books to be valuable sources of information on LCD/VLCD and recommend everyone read them as well. After reading these books, I knew that I had to try Dr. Bernstein's VLCD with a maximum of 30 grams carbohydrate/day to minimize hypoglycemia and the risk of developing long-term diabetic complications. I had the added perspective as a physician of seeing first-hand the actual consequences of having poorly-controlled diabetes. As a nephrologist, a specialist in kidney diseases, I took care of thousands of patients with diabetic nephropathy, the kidney disease caused by poor glycemic control. I had to start some of them on dialysis for end-stage kidney failure and managed their care for a wide range of other diabetic complications. In fact, in 1999, diabetes became the leading cause of kidney failure in the U.S. due to the rapid rise in the number of persons with T2D. My job was to help those with diabetic nephropathy improve their glycemic control to prevent worsening of kidney function and CVD, the leading cause of death in those with T1D and T2D. CVD in those with diabetes results from hyperglycemia, glycemic variability, hyperinsulinemia (elevated insulin levels in the blood), systemic inflammation, and arterial wall plaque deposition. When an arterial plaque ruptures, the clotting that results can block the artery, causing heart attack, stroke, sudden death, or lower extremity gangrene leading to limb amputation.

Beginning the Very Low-Carbohydrate Diet

On February 8, 2012, I started my VLCD which, in hindsight, was a new beginning in my life with T1D. Within days, my blood sugar excursions and the mealtime lispro (Humalog) doses began to decrease due to the replacement of dietary carbohydrate with fat. During the first three months on the VLCD, my mean blood glucose was 123 mg/dl (6.8 mM) (a 15% reduction compared to the Paleo Diet), SDBG was 49 mg/dl (2.7 mM) (a 38% reduction), COV was 40% (a 26% reduction), and the mean TDID was 20.3 IU/day or 0.30 IU/kg/day (a 47% reduction) at bodyweight of 67.7 kg (148.9 lb.). I also noticed that the frequency of hypoglycemia, hyperglycemia, and need for dextrose during exercise decreased significantly over time. This was likely due to the VLCD-induced increase in muscular fatty acid utilization which specifically inhibits the rate of muscular glucose utilization; called the glucose/fatty acid cycle first described in 1963 [Dimitriadis, G, et al., 2011]. As a result of these improvements, I felt more confident that I could safely do an ironman-distance triathlon with reasonably good blood sugar control. On October 20, 2012, I completed an ironman-distance triathlon with no untoward events. My blood glucose readings were mildly elevated throughout the event as a result of omitting my breakfast insulin dose to avoid hypoglycemia. My blood glucose peaked at about 200 mg/dl (11.1 mM) after the 2.4 mile swim and gradually decreased during the 112-mile bike and 26.2-mile marathon. My blood glucose after crossing the finish line was ≈ 150 mg/dl (≈ 8.3 mM), 15.5 hours after the start. I never experienced hypoglycemia and did not need to consume any food or dextrose. With plans to do another ironman-distance triathlon the following spring, I resumed training immediately. Yet another of my many training mistakes. I should have cut way back on my training so I could fully recover before preparing for the next event. Over the next several months, I developed plantar fasciosis in both feet from excessive training. This injury limited my ability to train and put a stop to my triathlons. During 2013 and 2014, I did less aerobic exercise and added more resistance exercise. I enjoyed doing less training and found my blood sugar was better controlled with shorter exercise sessions. It took almost three years for the plantar fasciosis to completely resolve and I decided not to do any more triathlons.

In 2013, my mean blood glucose was 95 mg/dl (5.3 mM), SDBG was 40 mg/dl (2.2 mM), COV was 42%, and TDID was 28.3 IU. I switched my bolus insulin back to Humulin R again per Dr. Bernstein's protocol, but found my 3-hour post-meal blood glucose was consistently higher compared to using lispro (Humalog). I switched back to lispro (Humalog) and continue using it today. I explain in Chapter 5 why some with T1D have success with rapid-acting insulin analogs on a LCD, while others do better with short-acting regular insulin. In 2014, I decided to lower my blood glucose target to 83 mg/dl (4.6 mM) per Dr. Bernstein's protocol. My average blood glucose was 85 mg/dl (4.7 mM), SDBG was 35 mg/dl (1.9 mM), COV was 41%, and TDID was 31.5 IU. This reduction in average blood glucose required more insulin and resulted in significantly more hypoglycemia, albeit asymptomatic most of the time, due to hypoglycemia unawareness (see Chapter 10).

In September 2014, I closed my solo private practice allowing me to focus on achieving optimal health and helping those with diabetes to better control their diabetes via writing articles and books and online coaching at https://ketogenicdiabeticathlete.wordpress.com/coaching/. This is my third book on diabetes and I plan to continue writing and updating them as new information becomes available. In March 2015, I started olympic weightlifting which is both enjoyable and challenging at the same time. My current exercise regimen consists of daily olympic weightlifting and a daily walk and gardening outdoors. It has taken several years to sort out the exact type, intensity, frequency, and volume of exercises from which I can recover by the next day to avoid overtraining. My current exercise regimen consumes considerably less time than the triathlon training I did for five years. The regularity and consistency of daily walking and resistance training has improved my glycemic variability due to more stable insulin sensitivity compared to intermittent long-distance triathlon training.

Physical activity is essential for a healthy life, just like healthful eating. The maximal benefits of exercise will not be realized unless done regularly. Exercise results in an overall feeling of well-being and has numerous long-term health benefits. For those with diabetes, exercise has direct beneficial effects due to improved insulin sensitivity, increased lean muscle mass, improved body composition, and reduced insulin doses. In Chapter 7, I review the benefits of exercise and the strategies I have developed to improve blood sugar management with exercise.

In 2015, I increased my target blood glucose to reduce the frequency of hypoglycemia. My average blood glucose was 95 mg/dl (5.3 mM), SDBG was 37 mg/dl (2.1 mM), COV was 39%, mean TDID was 31.8 IU, and I had fewer hypoglycemic blood glucose readings. In 2016, my blood sugar statistics were almost identical to 2015. In 2017, I succeeded in gaining weight from 70 kg (154 lb.) to 75 kg (165 lb.) as I was aiming for the 77 kg (169.4 lb.) bodyweight class in olympic weightlifting. My average blood glucose was 99 mg/dl (5.5 mM), SDBG was 43 mg/dl (2.4 mM), COV was 43%, and TDID was 36.7 IU. My insulin requirements increased as a result of gaining weight. I was still not satisfied with my glycemic control and variability and wanted to further reduce the frequency of hypoglycemia. It has been hypothesized that variation in blood glucose in combination with HbA1c, may be a more reliable indicator of one's risk for long-term complications than is mean HbA1c alone [Soupal, J, et al., 2014]. Briefly, the authors postulated that increased variation in blood sugar would generate more reactive oxygen species (ROS) in complication-prone cells due to hyperglycemia-induced oxidative stress [Hirsch, IB, et al., 2005, King, GL, et al., 2004]. This overproduction of ROS by the mitochondrial electron-transport chain contributes to glucose-mediated vascular damage, i.e., atherosclerosis. The mitochondria are small organelles in most cells that produce most of the adenosine triphosphate (ATP) we need to fuel every chemical reaction in the body. The electron-transport chain is a series of enzymes inside the mitochondria which create a proton (H$^+$) gradient across the inner mitochondrial membrane to power the production of ATP by ATP synthase.

In 2018, the International Weightlifting Federation changed all of the weight classes for competition in olympic weightlifting. My bodyweight had peaked at 75 kg (165 lb.), so I decided to aim for 73 kg (160.6 lb.) or 67 kg (147.4 lb.). I simply eliminated the lunch that I had added to gain weight. After eliminating lunch for a month, my bodyweight was 71 kg (156.2 lb.), so I decided to see if I could get down to 67 kg (147.4 lb.). I used cronometer.com to design my meals using a macronutrient intake of ≤ 50 grams of total carbohydrate, ≈ 2.3 grams/kg/day of protein, and I reduced my dietary fat intake to lose more body fat while still meeting 100% of the recommended daily allowance (RDA) for all the micronutrients (vitamins and minerals). Over several months, I slowly reduced my dietary fat in 200 kcal/day (22 grams/day of dietary fat) steps to reduce my bodyweight to 67 kg (147.4 lb.). By the time I reached 67 kg (147.4 lb.), I had developed several symptoms of insufficient caloric intake including generalized fatigue, feeling cold, increasing thoughts of food, but interestingly, no hunger, possibly an effect of my higher-protein ketogenic VLCD. I knew a 67 kg (147.4 lb.) bodyweight would be unsustainable in the long-term, so I decided to go back up to 73 kg (160.6 lb.) where I have remained since. As I lost bodyweight, I had to lower my insulin doses and then increase them again as I regained bodyweight. For the month of May 2019, my average blood glucose was 103 mg/dl (5.7 mM), SDBG was 30 mg/dl (1.7 mM), COV was 29%, and mean TDID was 18.7 IU at a bodyweight of 67.3 kg (148 lb.) or 0.28 IU/kg/day demonstrating that both total bodyweight and % body fat (I was quite lean) are significant determinants of TDID [Polonsky, KS, et al., 1988].

Can Lifestyle Consistency Result in Normal Blood Sugars?

I had always know that exogenous insulin was one source of glycemic variability that could not be completely eliminated. The medical literature suggested that day-to-day variation in insulin action was a significant, if not the primary, source of blood sugar variability. A recent review article [Gradel, AKJ, et al., 2018] stated that, "Variability in the subcutaneous absorption and effect of insulin represents an important source of glucose variability in patients using insulin and is thus a major challenge in insulin therapy." But I felt there had to be additional sources of glycemic variability and I was determined to find a method to further reduce the frequency of asymptomatic hypoglycemia. I decided to test the hypothesis that variation in lifestyle factors was the primary cause of my blood sugar variability. I thought if I could identify and correct all of these lifestyle factors, I could finally normalize my blood sugars. This would also minimize the frequency and associated risks of hypoglycemia and the potential to develop long-term diabetic complications. I decided to devise a more precise method of quantifying my meals and exercise regimen to minimize or eliminate all the variables that could be affecting my glycemic control. To increase my bodyweight back to 73 kg (160.6 lb.), I had already returned to three meals/day, each of which would now have a constant dietary protein, carbohydrate, and fat content while keeping the mealtimes constant as well: 7 AM, 12:30 PM, and 6 PM. I adjusted my exercise regimen multiple times to find a set of olympic weightlifting exercises that I could recover from by the following day and result in normal post-exercise blood sugars. My exercise is performed at about the same time each day such that the insulin-sensitizing effect will be automatically factored into the corresponding bolus insulin dose (BID). I also started taking a BID at bedtime (10:30 PM), if needed, to correct for above-target blood sugar readings while keeping my bedtime basal insulin dose as constant as possible. I also adopted a more regimented sleep schedule as described in Chapter 8.

Blood Sugars in Healthy Humans

To understand what exactly 'normal blood sugars' are, I will present five publications from the medical literature which measured interstitial glucose (IG) with CGM in metabolically-healthy, nondiabetic subjects. A

CGM has a tiny probe that is inserted through the skin where it is bathed by the 'interstitial fluid' under the skin. This interstitial fluid 'leaks' out of the tiny blood vessels that course through the skin. The probe has an electronic sensor that measures the IG concentration every 5 mins. The IG reading is ideally the same as blood glucose except delayed by ≈ 15 mins.

The subjects in the five studies were confirmed to be metabolically-healthy using a medical history, physical exam, and extensive laboratory testing. The subjects were not taking any medications, had normal bodyweight, blood pressure, fasting blood glucose, HbA1c, fasting insulin and/or C-peptide levels, homeostatic model assessment of insulin resistance (HOMA-IR), and oral glucose tolerance tests (OGTT). HOMA-IR is simply the fasting insulin level multiplied by the fasting blood glucose. If either value are slightly elevated, then the product of the two will be elevated and is an indication of insulin resistance, a precursor to diabetes. The OGTT measures several blood glucose values after consuming a 75-gram dextrose solution. If any of the values exceed a predetermined level, this too is indicative of insulin resistance, pre-diabetes, or diabetes. Subjects with any abnormal results were excluded from the studies below.

In the first of five studies [Freckmann, G, et al., 2007], the 24-hour IG was measured in 24 healthy nondiabetic volunteers (12 female, 12 male, age 27.1 years) using two CGM devices for two days while the subjects consumed self-selected diets at home with an average carbohydrate intake of 253 grams/day. The mean 24-hour IG was 89 mg/dl (5.0 mM) and the mean 24-hour blood glucose was 91 mg/dl (5.1 mM). This first study found that meals with fast-acting (high glycemic index) versus slow-acting carbohydrates (lower glycemic index), with identical carbohydrate content, resulted in higher peak post-meal IG, 122 mg/dl (6.8 mM) versus

99 mg/dl (5.5 mM), in the nondiabetic individuals. Thus you can see that the type of carbohydrate, in addition to the total amount of carbohydrate, determines the post-meal blood glucose response. This is called the glycemic load: the product of glycemic index and total carbohydrate intake. I wanted to use this study to not only illustrate normal blood sugar levels in nondiabetic subjects, but to also illustrate the concepts of glycemic index and load [Wolever, TMS, et al., 1991]. I will teach you how to formulate a LCD using foods with both low-glycemic indices and low-glycemic loads so as to minimize the rise in your post-meal blood sugar in Chapter 4.

In the second of five studies [Mazze, RS, et al., 2008], subjects with and without diabetes were recruited to participate in a prospective observational study employing CGM for 28 days. The mean IG for the 32 nondiabetic subjects was 102 mg/dl (5.7 mM) with a median standard deviation of interstitial glucose (SDIG) equal to 18 mg/dl (1.0 mM). The nondiabetic subjects were compared to individuals with diabetes representing the wide range of blood sugar control typically seen in clinical practice. The diabetic subjects included 15 subjects with T1D and 15 with T2D whose mean IG was 159 mg/dl (8.8 mM) and the median SDIG was 57 mg/dl (3.2 mM).

In the third of five studies [Beck, RW, et al., 2010], 74 nondiabetic children, adolescents, and adults aged 9–65 years used a blinded CGM device for 3–7 days. IG was slightly higher in children than in adults. For all 74 healthy subjects, the mean IG was 98 mg/dl (5.4 mM) and median SDIG was 13.7 mg/dl (0.76 mM). Analysis by age group is shown in Table 2.1.

Table 2.1 — Mean and Standard Deviation of IG by Age

Age Range (years) Number of Subjects (n)	Mean IG (mg/dl)	Mean IG (mM)	SDIG (mg/dl)	SDIG (mM)
8 to < 15, n = 20	103	5.72	16.4	0.91
15 to < 25, n = 17	97	5.39	13.7	0.76
25 to < 45, n = 20	96	5.33	12.6	0.70
≥ 45, n = 17	95	5.28	12.4	0.69

In the fourth of five studies [Zhou, J, et al., 2009], IG by CGM and blood glucose by finger-stick, four times daily, were measured for three days in 434 nondiabetic male and female subjects, age 20–69 years old, at 10 academic hospitals throughout China. The subject's meals were monitored and the total caloric intake from the three daily meals was 30 kcal/kg/day, with 50% of calories from carbohydrate, 15% from protein, and 35% from fat. When IG values and finger-stick blood glucose readings were simultaneously measured, the means were identical: 103 mg/dl (5.7 mM). Pearson correlation analysis revealed a positive correlation between IG values and finger-stick blood glucose readings (r = 0.822, P < 0.001). For the 434 healthy subjects, the mean 24-hour IG was 104 mg/dl (5.8 mM) and the median SDIG was 14 mg/dl (0.8 mM). The 95th percentile of mean 24-hour IG was 119 mg/dl (6.6 mM) which the authors considered to be normal.

The last study [Zhou, J, et al., 2011] presented statistics on the variation in IG as measured by the SDIG on the same 434 nondiabetic Chinese subjects just reviewed. The median SDIG was 13.5 (0.75 mmol/L). The 95th percentile of the SDIG was 25.2 mg/dl (1.40 mM) which the authors considered to be normal. The authors concluded that, "The values established in this study may facilitate the adoption of glycemic variability as a metric of overall glycemic control in diabetes." The results of all five studies are summarized in Table 2.2.

Table 2.2 — Mean and Standard Deviation of IG from Five Studies

Unit of measure for glycemic results	Mean IG, 5 studies, n = 564	95th percentile of mean IG, 1 study, n = 434	Median SDIG, 4 studies, n = 540	95th percentile of SDIG, 1 study, n = 434
mg/dl	89–104	119	13.5–18	25.2
mM	4.9–5.8	6.6	0.75–1.00	1.40

Finally Achieving Normal Blood Sugars

As of September 2019, I was able to achieve normal blood sugars like those of metabolically-healthy nondiabetics for the first time since my diagnosis in 1998! My average blood glucose was 101 mg/dl (5.6 mM), SDBG was 24 mg/dl (1.3 mM), COV was 24%, and mean TDID was 26.6 IU at a bodyweight of 72.9 kg (160.4 lb.) or 0.36 IU/kg/day. My hypothesis was validated. Better late than never! Nevertheless, I was not finished. I set new goals with even less glycemic variability and hypoglycemia. My new goal is to keep all blood glucose reading between 70–130 mg/dl (3.9–7.2 mM) with no values < 70 mg/dl (3.9 mM). My goal mean blood glucose remains at 100 mg/dl (5.6 mM), although a mean blood glucose ≤ 119 mg/dl (6.6 mM) would be normal as well. My goal SDBG is anywhere in the range 13.5–18 mg/dl (0.75–1.00 mM), although a SDBG ≤ 25.2 mg/dl (1.40 mM) would be normal as well. My goals are summarized in Table 2.3. Your target blood glucose should be set by you and your physician so that you will safely avoid hypoglycemia. In an effort to further improve my glycemic variation, I changed my basal insulin from glargine (Lantus) to degludec (Tresiba) on Nov. 22, 2019. I continued to improve my glycemic variability (SDBG), but it is difficult to know how much of the improvement was due to degludec (Tresiba) vs. other small refinements that I periodically made to my strategies. I was able to achieve the new SDBG goal as of January 2020.

Table 2.3 — Dr. Runyan's Blood Glucose Goals

Units	Target blood glucose	Goal blood glucose range	Monthly goal mean blood glucose	Monthly goal SDBG
mg/dl	100	70–130	98–104	13.5–18
mM	5.6	3.9–7.2	5.4–5.8	0.75–1.0

For me, consistency in diet, exercise, and sleep were the last additions that resulted in normal blood sugars with infrequent hypoglycemia and the peace of mind that I can live a normal life without diabetic complications. I recognize that the lifestyle changes I advocate in this book may seem extreme, impractical, or unnecessary and may not be easy to implement at first. I have to admit when I first heard about Dr. Bernstein's 30-gram/day VLCD, I thought it was extreme! But as I mentioned, I absolutely abhor hypoglycemia and was highly motivated to fix it. As I guide you through the details, I will provide alternatives to consider that might be more acceptable or doable with school, work, and family to consider as well. Nevertheless, I know there will be others, like me, who are fed-up with experiencing hypoglycemia and are willing to do whatever it takes to live a normal life. A life without the constant threat of another hypoglycemic episode, the pain and suffering of diabetic complications, and the early death that results. My suggestion is to review all of the changes I advocate with your physician, adopt them into your lifestyle at your own pace, assess the value of the benefits, and only then, judge whether or not to sustain them. You may find, as I did, that the benefits are well worth the necessary lifestyle changes. Once you adapt to the new lifestyle, I expect you will find that the changes are neither burdensome, nor difficult.

I post my blood sugar results every month on my blog at https://ketogenicdiabeticathlete.wordpress.com and have done so since November 2015.

3 – Erratic Blood Sugars in Type 1 Diabetes

"Variability is the law of life, … and no two individuals react alike and behave alike under the abnormal conditions which we know as disease."
Sir William Osler, MDCM, a founding father of modern medicine, Johns Hopkins University.

"There's a way to do it better — find it."
Thomas Edison, America's greatest inventor.

"Where there is a will, there is a way."
Pauline Kael, American Critic & Author

The Bleak State of Glycemic Control in Type 1 Diabetes

If you have had T1D for even a short time, you know that blood sugar is exceedingly difficult to regulate. In fact, the average HbA1c among 16,061 persons in the T1D Exchange Clinic Registry was 8.4% as of 2014 [Miller, KM, et al., 2015]. This is roughly equivalent to an average blood glucose of 222 mg/dl (12.3 mM) [Rohlfing, CL, et al., 2002]. Most with T1D also have abnormally high glycemic variability. Both elevated average blood sugar and glycemic variability explain why those with T1D experience, 1) recurrent hypoglycemia, 2) develop long-term complications of diabetes [Brownlee, M, et al., 2006], and 3) a reduction in lifespan of 11–13 years [Livingstone, SJ, et al., 2015]. In this study [Foster, NC, et al., 2019], data on T1D management and outcomes from 22,697 registry participants (age 1–93 years) were collected in 2016–2018 and compared with data collected in 2010–2012 for 25,529 registry participants.

Insulin pump use increased from 57% in 2010–2012 to 63% in 2016–2018. CGM use increased from 7% in 2010–2012 to 30% in 2016–2018. Despite these increases, mean glycemic control as measured by HbA1c did not improve, but instead deteriorated, as shown in Table 3.1.

Table 3.1 — State of Glycemic Control in T1D

	Age < 6	Age 6-12	Age 13-17	Age 18-25	Age 26-49	Age ≥ 50
HbA1c, 2010-2012	8.1%	8.4%	8.5%	8.4%	7.6%	7.6%
HbA1c, 2016-2018	8.4%	8.6%	9.0%	8.8%	7.7%	7.7%
% Using CGM, 2010-2012	4%	3%	3%	4%	15%	15%
% Using CGM, 2016-2018	51%	37%	24%	22%	37%	34%

In this chapter, I will review the major sources of erratic blood sugars in those with T1D. The good news is that most can be minimized or eliminated with a better understanding of, 1) why a low-fat high-carbohydrate diet (LFHCD) causes erratic blood sugars, 2) how exogenous insulin works differently than endogenous β-cell insulin, and 3) how physical activity and exercise influence one's response to exogenous insulin.

Why a LFHCD Causes Erratic Blood Sugars

Of all the lifestyle choices we can make, diet has the most impact on our blood sugar control. Although most of us with T1D were instructed to follow a LFHCD by our well-meaning diabetes care team, the LFHCD is the major source of erratic blood sugars in those with diabetes and is simply not compatible with normal blood sugar control! Your diabetes care team is not aware that the LFHCD was based on a hypothesis that dietary fat contributed to CVD, but when actually tested, was never found to be true [Harcombe, Z, et al., 2016]. The 'experts' promoting the hypothesis suffered from cognitive dissonance and continued to promote it despite evidence to the contrary. I believe your diabetes care team has noble intentions and are relying on experts who, unfortunately, did not follow the scientific method in arriving at their dietary recommendations for T1D. Because of the LFHCD, persons with T1D have erratic blood sugars and medical practitioners just assume that this is the normal state of T1D. They are, at best, simply trying to help you reach a HbA1c in the 6.5–7% range or a 140–154 mg/dl (7.8–8.6 mM) average blood glucose in adults and 7.5% HbA1c or a 168 mg/dl (9.3 mM) average blood glucose in children and adolescents. They know diabetic complications can occur and their job is to detect and treat them with various medications and procedures. I prescribed diabetes and blood pressure medications to my patients and ordered dialysis treatments for many years without knowing that their diabetic complications were preventable with different dietary and lifestyle choices. But as I pointed out in Chapter 2, the only effective solution is to address the root cause and either prevent the diabetic complications or reverse them by normalizing blood sugars. When a T1D patient's HbA1c is < 6.5%, the practitioner's first concern will be that the patient is having frequent episodes of hypoglycemia. This is an appropriate concern when the patient is following a LFHCD. But when following a LCD, one must examine the mean blood glucose or IG, glycemic variability as measured by SDBG or SDIG, and the frequency of hypoglycemic episodes to properly assess glycemic control. Simply measuring HbA1c is a blunt tool as will be discussed in Chapter 6.

Given that the LFHCD causes erratic blood sugars and is more likely a cause of CVD than a preventive measure, it makes more sense to normalize our blood sugars utilizing a LCD [Feinman, RD, et al., 2015]. This is due to the simple fact that of all the dietary macronutrients, persons with diabetes are the most intolerance of carbohydrates. **Put simply, diabetes is a state of dietary carbohydrate intolerance.** The reality is, in order to have normal blood sugars the vast majority of the time, persons with T1D must follow a dietary regimen that minimizes post-meal blood glucose excursions: the LCD is one such dietary pattern. A Mediterranean-style diet, plant-based diet, vegetarian diet, carnivore diet, Paleo diet and many others could be effective as well, as long as processed foods, sugars, refined-carbohydrates, and vegetable oils are excluded and the total daily carbohydrate intake does not exceed 100 grams/day.

To fully understand why a LFHCD leads to erratic blood sugars, you need to know a little bit about how the body handles the food you eat and the role insulin plays in that process. Food is a mixture of macronutrients (protein, carbohydrate, and fat) and micronutrients (vitamins and minerals). Digestion of nutrients in a meal involves physical, chemical, and enzymatic processes. In the mouth, chewing breaks up food physically and amylase in the saliva is an enzyme that cleaves starches into sugar; glucose to be exact. Glucose is the sugar that we measure when checking our blood sugar. We haven't even made it past the mouth and you already know why starches from wheat, corn, oats, potato, bread, rice, pasta and cereals raise blood sugar so quickly. After swallowing your chewed food and drink, the stomach physically churns the mixture and secretes hydrochloric acid (HCl), pepsin, intrinsic factor, and mucus. The HCl breaks chemical bonds in the food, the enzyme, pepsin, cleaves proteins into amino acids only in the acidic environment created by HCl, intrinsic factor facilitates the absorption of vitamin B12 in the ileum (the first segment of the colon), and the mucus protects the stomach lining from the HCl.

After passing through the stomach, partially digested food enters the duodenum where secretions from both the gallbladder and the exocrine pancreas are added. The pancreas makes sodium bicarbonate (baking soda) that serves to neutralize the HCl that emptied into the duodenum from the stomach. The pancreas also makes multiple enzymes that digest protein, carbohydrates, and fat. The enzymes trypsin, chymotrypsin, and carboxypolypeptidase break down proteins to form amino acids. Pancreatic amylase, the same enzyme in saliva, cleaves starch into glucose. The enzyme pancreatic lipase cleaves fat (triglycerides) into fatty acids and monoglycerides (glycerol bound to one fatty acid). The exocrine pancreatic secretions are mixed with bile salts that are synthesized by the liver and stored in the gallbladder which is located adjacent to the liver. Bile salts are not enzymes, but are useful for two functions: they help to emulsify the large fat particles in the food into many tiny particles, the surface of which can then be accessed by pancreatic lipase and secondly can aid in the absorption of the digested fat through the intestinal mucosal membrane. Those who have had their gallbladder removed (cholecystectomy) usually have no problem digesting fat on a LCD because the liver actually makes the bile salts. Bile also functions to remove waste products from the blood including bilirubin (from hemoglobin degradation) and cholesterol. The digested food then passes into the small intestine where amino acids, simple sugars (fructose, lactose, galactose, and glucose), and fatty acids are absorbed into the bloodstream. These nutrients also stimulate secretion of two incretins, glucagon-like peptide–1 (GLP-1) and glucose-dependent insulinotropic peptide (GIP), by the intestinal cells which magnify β-cell insulin secretion in response to blood glucose, inhibit α-cell glucagon secretion, and slow gastric emptying. Due to the lack of β-cells in those with T1D, these incretins only serve to slow gastric emptying to help mitigate the post-meal rise in blood glucose [Marathe, CS, et al., 2011].

Amino acids from the protein eaten in a meal are used to synthesize new proteins which compose structural components of cells, enzymes that catalyze all the biochemical reactions in the body, membrane transport molecules, receptors, and many hormones, e.g., insulin, amylin, and glucagon to name a few. Tissue proteins are recycled daily and some is used to make adenosine triphosphate (ATP), the universal fuel for all cells, or converted to glucose, fat, or ketones per the body's needs. Fatty acids from the fat eaten in a meal are used as a fuel to make ATP and along with cholesterol, make up a large portion of the structural components of cell membranes (the lipid bilayer), organelles, and lipoproteins that transport triglycerides and cholesterol throughout the body. Fatty acids are stored in muscle and fat cells after combining with glycerol to form triglycerides for future use when we are not eating. Glucose, from the carbohydrate eaten in a meal as well as that made by the liver and kidneys, can be used by all tissues as a fuel to make ATP. Some glucose is used to make a wide variety of other compounds, e.g., glycerol, DNA, RNA and coenzymes like NAD$^+$ and NADH. Glucose destined to be used as fuel can be stored in limited quantities in the liver and muscles as glycogen. Glycogen in mammals is analogous to starch in plants. Both are long chains of glucose molecules, but differ only by the specific type of linkages between the glucose molecules. The liver can store a total of ≈ 100–125 grams of glycogen which can be converted back to glucose via glycogenolysis and released into the bloodstream when needed. This process is stimulated by lower insulin and higher glucagon concentrations in the blood. Skeletal muscle can store a total of ≈ 400–600 grams of glycogen that can be converted back to glucose and used to fuel the muscles. The glycogen in muscles is not a potential source of glucose for the purpose of raising blood sugar as it is in the liver. The liver (and kidneys only during prolonged fasting) makes new glucose molecules (gluconeogenesis) from the 18 glucogenic amino acids, pyruvate, lactate, glycerol (from triglycerides), and even acetone (one of the three ketones) [Kaleta, C, et al., 2011]. The liver is capable of making all the glucose the body needs without eating carbohydrates. **Thus, even though glucose is an essential nutrient, it is not essential that we consume it in our diet. Those with T1D can make use of this physiological fact by minimizing the one nonessential dietary macronutrient that causes the greatest excursion in our post-meal blood sugar — carbohydrate!**

Those with T1D are taught to count carbohydrates in a meal as a means to determine BID. This is a flawed method for several reasons. The amount of dietary carbohydrate consumed in a meal is more inaccurate than one might imagine. This is because the data on the Nutrition Facts Label or in nutrition databases is not independently verified or regulated, i.e., the U.S. Food and Drug Administration (FDA) relies upon the food industry to accurately report the nutrition data, but does not independently test anything. More importantly, the glycemic load is also affected by many other factors including whether it is raw or cooked, the temperature of the food when eaten, the other foods in the meal with which it is eaten, none of which can be accurately predicted. The larger the carbohydrate content of a meal, the larger the required BID, and the larger the potential mismatch between the two. This combined with variability in insulin sensitivity due to day-to-day changes in lifestyle factors, results in potentially large deviations in the post-meal blood sugar from one's target. This is why including a significant amount of carbohydrates in the diet and attempting to count them is so ineffective for those with T1D. This study [Bao, J, et al., 2009] found that, "The relative insulin demand evoked by mixed meals is best predicted by a physiologic index based on actual insulin responses to isoenergetic portions of single foods." The authors concluded that, "In the context of composite meals of similar energy value but varying macronutrient content, carbohydrate counting was of limited value." Many years ago, I personally spent two years weighing my food and counting carbohydrates with no significant improvement in my glycemic control. I suppose I persisted in this futile attempt because I lacked an alternative approach at the time.

Insulin, Amylin, and Glucagon Keep Blood Sugars Normal

Normally, blood sugar is maintained in a narrow range by the ability of the pancreatic β-cells to vary insulin and amylin secretion and the neighboring alpha-cells (α-cells) to vary glucagon secretion in response to the prevailing blood glucose concentration. Insulin is an anabolic hormone that facilitates, 1) the transport of glucose into cells by signaling for the insertion additional glucose transporters (GLUT4) into cell membranes, 2) the synthesis of proteins from amino acids, 3) the synthesis glycogen from glucose, storing it for later use, 4) the conversion of glucose to fatty acids (de novo lipogenesis) by the liver and fat cells, and 5) the uptake of fatty acids into fat cells and their storage as triglycerides. Insulin also 6) inhibits glucagon secretion by the α-cells, 7) inhibits liver glucose production via glycogenolysis and gluconeogenesis, 8) inhibits the release of fatty acids from fat cells, and 9) inhibits the synthesis and release of ketones by the liver. Amylin assists insulin by suppressing glucagon secretion by the α-cells, slowing stomach emptying, and promoting satiety, all of which reduce the post-meal increase in blood glucose. Glucagon, on the other hand, is a catabolic hormone that stimulates, 1) the breakdown of liver glycogen to make glucose (glycogenolysis), 2) the synthesis of new glucose (gluconeogenesis), 3) the release of fatty acids from fat cells, and 4) the synthesis of ketones by the liver [Liljenquist, JE, et al., 1974]. The levels of insulin and amylin around the α-cell regulates its glucagon secretion. Low insulin and amylin levels, when not eating, stimulate glucagon secretion, whereas high insulin and amylin levels, while eating meals, suppress glucagon secretion to maintain normal blood glucose levels around the clock. The presence of amino acids from dietary protein stimulates both insulin, and to a greater extent, glucagon secretion in nondiabetics which serves to prevent hypoglycemia after a high-protein low-carbohydrate meal, e.g., a steak. And as mentioned previously, the incretins, GLP-1 and GIP, magnify β-cell insulin secretion and inhibit α-cell glucagon secretion. These hormones, working together, maintain appropriate blood glucose, lipid, and ketone levels by storing and releasing nutrients to provide a continuous supply of energy to our body around the clock: after meals, between meals, during exercise, and while fasting.

Injected Insulin is Not Equivalent to β-Cell Insulin

The insulin preparations used to treat T1D do not exactly replicate the insulin-secreting capability of normal pancreatic β-cells described above. No doubt we are very fortunate to have a wide variety of insulin options including basal and bolus insulin preparations administered via injection and pump. Although treating T1D with exogenous insulin is necessary and life-saving, it is responsible for some of the erratic blood sugar responses that follow. There are five sources of glycemic variability related to exogenous insulin: 1) mismatch between rate of appearance of exogenous insulin in the bloodstream (a function of the insulin preparation being used) and the rate of nutrient absorption (due to amylin deficiency, diabetic gastroparesis, and the macronutrient composition of the meal), 2) day-to-day variability in insulin action (a function of the insulin preparation being used), 3) the injection location and technique affect the rate of insulin absorption and action, 4) insulin is absorbed into the bloodstream from the site of injection irrespective of the current blood glucose concentration, and 5) the inherent mismatch that results from injecting exogenous insulin into the subcutaneous fat (under the skin) rather than being released by the β-cells. Understanding why exogenous insulin differs from insulin made and secreted by the β-cells helps us to manage T1D more effectively. The first three sources of blood sugar variability due to insulin can be minimized with an understanding of the properties of the different insulin preparations and proper insulin injection technique, both covered in Chapter 5. The last two sources of glycemic variability stem from the differences between insulin secreted by the β-cells and exogenous insulin. The two main differences are: 1) endogenous insulin is secreted on a minute-by-minute basis by the β-cells inside the pancreas according to the prevailing blood glucose level and other hormonal and macronutrient influences, whereas exogenous insulin diffuses into the peripheral blood circulation from the site of injection according to its chemical properties as designed by the manufacturer regardless of the current blood glucose concentration and 2) the endogenous insulin concentration surrounding the α-cells is 100-times, and that reaching the liver, is 3-times higher than in the rest of the body, whereas exogenous insulin used in those with T1D has the same concentration throughout the entire body [Unger, RH, et al., 2012]. In addition, the enhancement of β-cell insulin secretion by the incretins, GLP-1 and GIP, does not occur in those with T1D. These differences explain why exogenous insulin does not properly control glucagon secretion and liver glucose production especially after meals. This can lead to exaggerated post-meal blood glucose responses and chronically elevated glucagon levels and liver glucose production in those with T1D especially in the setting of insulin deficiency characterized by hyperglycemia [Hughes, DS, et al., 2014, Müller, WA, et al., 1971] as well as insulin resistance in muscle and fat tissues [Hager, SR, et al. 1991]. Thus, chronic hyperglycemia in T1D results in a state similar to that of T2D, i.e., insulin deficiency and insulin resistance.

In light of these facts, to normalize blood sugars, we must devise strategies to mitigate these problems. A LCD mitigates the post-meal rise in blood sugar as a result of its reduced carbohydrate (glucose) load. The post-meal increase in liver glucose production can also be diminished in those with T1D with the oral diabetes medication, metformin, as discussed in Chapter 11. Furthermore, muscle responds to regular exercise by taking up and utilizing glucose which helps mitigate the effects of chronically elevated liver glucose production as discussed in Chapter 7. Finally, by more closely matching insulin needs with precisely-dosed exogenous insulin as discussed in Chapter 5, we can avoid both hypoglycemia (and the subsequent counterregulatory hormone release that can cause insulin resistance and hyperglycemia) and hyperglycemia (and the subsequent increase in insulin resistance and increase in glucagon secretion from insulin deficiency). In other words, erratic blood sugars beget erratic blood sugars and normal blood sugars beget normal blood sugars and reduced TDID. We will aim for the later.

Exercise Influences the Response to Exogenous Insulin

Another important source of erratic blood sugars in those with T1D stems from physical activity and exercise. Physical activities like playing outside, doing chores around the house, physical jobs, exercise, or other activities, done on an irregular or spontaneous basis can result in the surprise of low or high blood sugars. Because the type, intensity, frequency, and duration of exercise affects muscle insulin sensitivity and counterregulatory hormone secretion to different extents, those with T1D need to understand these factors in order to make adjustments in insulin administration, and/or glucose (dextrose) supplementation, and/or exercise to prevent unwanted changes in, or to correct, blood sugars.

The blood sugar response to exercise is dependent on three main factors: 1) the current insulin-on-board, meaning how much insulin remains in the subcutaneous fat that has not yet diffused into the bloodstream, 2) the current muscle insulin sensitivity which is dependent on previous bouts of exercise, and 3) the type, duration, and intensity of exercise.

Insulin-on-Board

Insulin-on-board includes both bolus and basal insulin. Rapid-acting insulin analogs remain active for ≈ 5 hours and short-acting regular insulin for ≈ 8–10 hours after injection whereas basal insulin works continuously, but can vary somewhat during a 24-hour period. Depending on the timing of exercise, including time-of-day and time after a bolus insulin injection, the blood sugar response to exercise can vary significantly. Exercising soon after a bolus insulin injection can have a different effect on the blood sugar response to exercise compared to starting that same exercise several hours after the same bolus insulin injection. This is due, in part, to the exercise-induced increase in blood flow in the area of the insulin injection which hastens insulin absorption into the bloodstream. Exercise also diverts blood flow away from the intestines and can slow the absorption of nutrients. This combined effect of exercise on insulin and nutrient absorption explains the different blood sugar responses to exercise based on the timing of the exercise relative to a meal and its accompanying bolus insulin injection.

Basal insulin is continuously diffusing from each site of injection into the bloodstream for several days. The amount of insulin released from any given injection site varies with time. The dose of basal insulin is a significant factor in the blood sugar response to exercise. Too little basal insulin being released during exercise can result in high blood sugar and too much basal insulin can result in hypoglycemia. The time of basal insulin injection also affects blood sugar over the next 24 hours and varies with the particular basal insulin preparation. Thus, factors that influence, or can be adjusted to compensate for exercise-related blood glucose fluctuations include: 1) the basal insulin preparation used, its dose, and timing of injection, or the insulin pump basal rate, 2) the mealtime bolus insulin preparation used, its dose, and timing of injection, before and after exercise, and 3) glucose (dextrose) supplementation, before, during, and after exercise.

Muscle Insulin Sensitivity

The blood glucose response to exercise is also influenced by exercise-induced improvements in muscle insulin sensitivity. Exercise improves muscular glucose uptake during, and for 2 hours after exercise, by a muscular contraction-dependent, insulin-independent, mechanism mediated by increased 5' adenosine monophosphate-activated protein kinase (AMPK) activity which promotes GLUT4 translocation, i.e., movement of glucose transport proteins, to the cell membrane and thereby increases cellular glucose uptake. "Studies assessing the acute responses during or immediately following a single bout of aerobic exercise suggest that insulin sensitivity is improved by more than 50% for up to 72 hours after the last exercise bout. However, this acute improvement in insulin sensitivity is lost within 5 days after the last exercise bout, even in highly trained subjects" [Bird, SR, 2017]. This improved muscle insulin sensitivity is not constant during the post-exercise period. In other words, if you exercise every 3 days (72 hours) do not assume your blood sugars will be easy to manage because your insulin sensitivity will be changing daily. Thus, irregular bouts of exercise is a source of erratic blood sugars due to changing insulin sensitivity. I personally experienced this from training for both triathlons and olympic weightlifting. Intermittent exercise, e.g., exercising some days, but not others, definitely leads to more erratic blood sugars than daily exercise, or dare I say, no exercise at all.

Type, Duration, and Intensity of Exercise

Different types, durations, and intensities of exercise have different effects on the post-exercise blood sugar. For example, endurance exercise when performed intermittently can result in hypoglycemia in those with T1D. In non-diabetics, endurance exercise suppresses insulin secretion which prevents hypoglycemia [Borghouts, LB, et al., 1999], but in T1D, exogenous insulin is unregulated and can result in hypoglycemia unless pre-exercise insulin doses are appropriately reduced or dextrose supplementation is taken. Conversely, high-intensity bouts of exercise when performed intermittently can result in hyperglycemia. The body can respond to high-intensity exercise by secreting counterregulatory hormones to assist in providing the muscles with additional fuel. These hormones include epinephrine, glucagon, cortisol, and growth hormone, all of which acutely raise blood sugar even in those without diabetes [Marliss, EB, et al., 2002, Thomas, F, et al., 2016]. Post-exercise hyperglycemia can be prevented with a regular schedule of exercise or corrected afterwards with a BID. Scheduling a meal after exercise allows the correction dose to be added to the BID. My self-experimentation with both endurance and resistance exercise revealed the best way to prevent hypoglycemia and hyperglycemia is to perform similar type, duration, and intensity of exercise daily at the same time each day. This way, the effect of the exercise is already incorporated into the basal and BID reducing the need for exercise-related dextrose supplementation. These and other aspects of exercise-related insulin dosing are covered in Chapters 5 and 7.

Other Factors That Cause Erratic Blood Sugars

Additional causes of erratic blood sugars in those with T1D include chronic stress, poor sleep hygiene, certain medications, hormones in menstruating females, and illnesses. Chronic stress results in increases in cortisol which reduces insulin sensitivity and raises blood sugar. Poor sleep hygiene increases appetite, cravings for sugar, insulin resistance, and thus, blood sugars. Some medications increase, while others decrease, blood sugar. Yet other medications can mask the symptoms of hypoglycemia. Acute illnesses, e.g., infections, increase stress hormones that in turn increase blood sugars. These topics are reviewed in more detail in Chapters 8 and 9.

4 – The Low-Carbohydrate Diet

"Let food be thy medicine and medicine be thy food."
Hippocrates, Greek physician and the father of Western medicine.

"It's a law of nature that you can't live on processed foods."
Timothy Noakes, MD, DSc, exercise scientist and physician.

"If man made it, don't eat it."
Jack LaLanne, America's first nationally recognized fitness advocate.

In this chapter, I will explain how to design a sustainable and nutritionally complete, low-carbohydrate diet (LCD) to facilitate normalization of blood sugars in those with T1D. Using a LCD for T1D also reduces the frequency of low blood sugars (hypoglycemia), variations in blood sugar (glycemic variability), and TDID. This reduction in insulin dosage facilitates shedding body fat that is present in about half of those with T1D [Mottalib, A, et al., 2017]. Reducing the amount of insulin one is exposed to over a lifetime is also important because "Hyperinsulinemia directly and indirectly contributes to a vast array of metabolic diseases including all inflammatory conditions, all vascular diseases, gestational and type 2 diabetes, NAFLD, obesity and certain cancers and dementias. The mechanisms include increased production of: insulin growth factor-1; reactive oxidative species and advanced glycation end-products (AGEs); and triglyceride and fatty acids. Hyperinsulinemia also directly and indirectly affects many other hormones and cytokine mechanisms including leptin, adiponectin, and estrogen" [Crofts, CAP, et al., 2015].

Origin of the Low-Fat and Low-Carbohydrate Diets

The LCD is not a recent fad or untested intervention. It was actually used as the primary treatment for T1D before the discovery of insulin in 1921. Elliott P. Joslin, MD, the first diabetes specialist in America and founder of the Joslin Diabetes Clinic, still in operation today, used a VLCD with 10 g carbohydrate (2.4% of energy), 75 g protein (17.8%), and 150 g fat (79.9%) per day (60 kg bodyweight, 2.47 ketogenic ratio defined below) to treat his patients with diabetes. Dr. Joslin's VLCD was published in, *The Principles and Practice of Medicine*, a medical textbook by Sir William Osler, MDCM, in 1892 [Osler, SW, 1920]. Dr. Osler was one of the four founding fathers of Johns Hopkins Medical School. After the discovery of insulin in 1921, the VLCD was less often utilized since insulin was thought to be the 'cure' for T1D. Instead, a diet with 20% of energy from dietary carbohydrate, 10% from protein, and 70% from fat was recommended until 1940 [Kiple, KF, et al., (Editor), 2000].

One of the first things I learned in 2011 when I began reading about nutrition was the origin of the LFHCD that I grew up eating. It turns out that the LFHCD was based on a hypothesis, championed by Ancel Keys, PhD, that dietary saturated fat caused CVD and that a LFHCD would lower the risk of developing CVD [Taubes, G, 2007]. This story was fascinating and irritating at the same time upon realizing that *The Dietary Guidelines for Americans*, first released in 1977, was solely based on this hypothesis, not scientific evidence. A hypothesis is a proposed explanation, made on the basis of limited evidence, as a starting point for further investigation. Amazingly, the LFHCD was not then, and has not since, been found to reduce the risk of CVD [Harcombe, Z, et al., 2016] and in some studies was found to increase the risk of cancer [Ravnskov, U, et al., 2014]. Only recently are Americans beginning to understand the mistake that was made and many are making efforts to move away from processed foods, sugar, refined grain products, and vegetable oils. In fact, the LFHCD is thought to be a major contributory cause of obesity, T2D, and the majority of the chronic diseases that afflict Americans and Westernized nations throughout the world. All of these chronic diseases have been increasing in prevalence ever since processed foods were introduced in the late 1800s and further promulgated by the dietary guidelines in 1977. This recent study [Araujo, J, et al., 2018] found that the proportion of metabolically healthy individuals in the U.S. is alarmingly small: about 12% of the U.S. population. If you are interested in learning more about this nutrition debacle, I recommend that you read four books that tell the story more eloquently than I am able to do here. The first book is *Good Calories, Bad Calories*, by Gary Taubes [Taubes, G, 2007], the second is, *The Case Against Sugar*, by Gary Taubes [Taubes, G, 2016], the third is, *The Big Fat Surprise*, by Nina Teicholz [Teicholz, N, 2010], and the fourth is, *Nutrition and Physical Degeneration*, by Weston A. Price, DDS. [Price, WA, 1939].

The American Diabetes Association (ADA) is responsible for introducing the LFHCD as a dietary plan for those with diabetes. From 1940 to 1970, the ADA recommended a diet with 40% of calories from dietary carbohydrate, 20% from protein, and 40% from fat. In 1971, the recommendation for the portion of calories from dietary carbohydrate was increased to $\geq 45\%$ with 20% from protein and $\leq 35\%$ from fat in the ADA publication, *Nutritional Recommendations and Principles for Individuals with Diabetes Mellitus*. In their report [Steinberg, D, et al., 1971], they wrote the following: "Important dietary concepts have developed during the last decade which require some alteration in long-held precepts. There no longer appears to be any need to restrict disproportionately the intake of carbohydrates in the diet of most diabetic patients. Increase of dietary carbohydrate, even to extremes, without increase of total calories, does not appear to increase insulin requirement in the insulin-treated diabetic patient. In the less severe typically obese diabetic, substitution of carbohydrate for fat does not appear to elevate fasting blood glucose or worsen glucose tolerance in response to standard glucose loads. However, some adult diabetic patients are prone to endogenous hypertriglyceridemia, one of the risk factors associated with atherosclerosis. This possibility should always be checked, since triglyceride levels may be sensitive to increases in dietary carbohydrate [see also: Ahrens, EH, et al., 1961]. The average proportion of calories consumed as carbohydrate in the U.S. population as a whole approximates 45 per cent; this proportion or even higher appears to be acceptable for the usual diabetic patient as well. It is not yet possible to obtain uniform agreement as to the optimal proportion of carbohydrate and fat calories recommended for the diabetic. The long-range effect of extreme changes, such as a high carbohydrate diet, on diabetic complications in a population not adapted to such diets is not known. On the other hand, a liberalized carbohydrate intake for the diabetic will necessarily be associated with a decrease in dietary fat and cholesterol. At the present time, there is not enough evidence to determine to what extent restriction of dietary fat and cholesterol is desirable. However, diabetic patients appear to respond to reduction of saturated fat and cholesterol intake with a lowering of circulating cholesterol, as do nondiabetic persons. There is at present no firm evidence that this restriction will retard the development of diabetic complications, particularly atherosclerosis. However, the epidemiologic and experimental evidence relating circulating lipids to atherosclerotic cardiovascular disease also appears to apply to the diabetic patient." There are numerous unsubstantiated statements and admissions of uncertainty in this quotation from the ADA that makes me question why any change in dietary recommendations was being made. No clinical trial had been conducted to determine its effect in those with diabetes. **The fact was then, and remains now, that diabetes is a state of carbohydrate intolerance.** Unfortunately, the ADA made a successful effort to promote these dietary recommendations widely and, in my opinion, harmed millions of people with diabetes in the process. In 1986, the recommended dietary carbohydrate intake for those with diabetes was again increased to ≤ 60% of energy, with 12–20% from protein and ≤ 30% from fat [Kiple, KF, et al., (Editor), 2000]. Despite this 80-year folly of recommending a LFHCD for the treatment of diabetes, the ADA has slowly shifted its position away from the LFHCD and now acknowledges the effectiveness of a LCD for diabetes. In the most recent 2020 ADA annual position statement titled, *Standards of Medical Care in Diabetes — 2020* [Riddle, MC, et al., 2020], the authors have reviewed the latest evidence for nutritional therapy for diabetes and now support the use of a LCD for diabetes. These statements include the following:

1. "Evidence suggests that there is not an ideal percentage of calories from carbohydrate, protein, and fat for people with diabetes. Therefore, macronutrient distribution should be based on an individualized assessment of current eating patterns, preferences, and metabolic goals [i.e., normal blood sugars].

2. The Mediterranean-style, low-carbohydrate, and vegetarian or plant-based eating patterns are all examples of healthful eating patterns that have shown positive results in research, but individualized meal planning should focus on personal preferences, needs, and goals.

3. Reducing overall carbohydrate intake for individuals with diabetes has demonstrated the most evidence for improving glycemia and may be applied in a variety of eating patterns that meet individual needs and preferences.

4. Until the evidence surrounding comparative benefits of different eating patterns in specific individuals strengthens, health care providers should focus on the key factors that are common among the patterns: 1) emphasize nonstarchy vegetables, 2) minimize added sugars and refined grains, and 3) choose whole-foods over highly-processed foods to the extent possible."

I believe these statements from the ADA should be enough to convince your diabetes care team that a LCD is appropriate for those with T1D.

Who Should Not Use a Low-Carbohydrate Diet

Before we get started designing a LCD, I need to let you know that there are some unusual medical conditions that are contraindications to using a LCD. These absolute contraindications include: carnitine deficiency (primary), carnitine palmitoyltransferase I or II deficiency, and carnitine translocase deficiency. There are five beta-oxidation defect syndromes: short-chain acyl dehydrogenase deficiency, medium-chain acyl dehydrogenase deficiency, long-chain acyl dehydrogenase deficiency, medium-chain 3-hydroxyacyl Co-A deficiency, long-chain 3-hydroxyacyl Co-A deficiency, and two additional conditions: pyruvate carboxylase deficiency and porphyria that are also absolute contraindications to using a LCD. Familial renal glycosuria is caused by a mutation in the gene for SGLT2 (sodium-glucose co-transporter-2) leads to excretion of glucose in the urine (glucouria). Persons with this genetic mutation are susceptible to ketoacidosis under conditions of stress, infection, and particularly during fasting or a LCD. These conditions are typically diagnosed in childhood by a pediatrician. You should check with your physician about these conditions prior to embarking on a LCD.

Those taking an SGLT2 inhibitor, canagliflozin (Invokana), dapagliflozin (Farxiga), empagliflozin (Jardiance), or ipragliflozin (currently only in Japan), should discuss its continued use before starting a LCD due to the potential risk for DKA (see Chapter 9). Persons with advanced chronic kidney disease (stages 3b–5) [Runyan, KR, 2019], liver cirrhosis, congestive heart failure, or any medical condition for that matter should also consult with their own physician prior to making any changes to their diet or medication regimen. Now on to the LCD, a key strategy for normalizing blood sugars in those with T1D.

The Low-Carbohydrate Diet for Type 1 Diabetes

A LCD contains 51–100 grams, while a VLCD contains ≤ 50 grams, but typically 20–50 grams, of total dietary carbohydrate/day. Consuming less than 20 grams of carbohydrate/day is possible and some may choose or need to do so due to food intolerances or insulin resistance, but it does limit the amount of nonstarchy vegetables, nuts, seeds, fruit, and dairy that can be included in the diet, along with the micronutrients they provide. The foods in your LCD/VLCD should have a low-glycemic index and load (low-GI). This meta-analysis [Thomas, D, et al., 2009] of 11 relevant RCT involving 402 participants concluded that a low-GI diet can improve glycemic control in diabetes without increasing hypoglycemic events. See Table 4.1 for some examples of low- versus high-glycemic index foods. Foods with high-glycemic indices and loads are especially harmful to those with diabetes due to the resulting hyperglycemia and endogenous conversion of glucose to fructose by aldose reductase the via the polyol pathway which leads to tissue glycation, formation of AGEs, long-term diabetic complications, high blood pressure, obesity, metabolic syndrome, and NAFLD [Johnson, RJ, et al., 2020, Lanaspa, MA, et al., 2013]. The majority of the foods you choose should be single-ingredient, whole foods, of high nutritive value, and preferably cooked at home [Wolfson, JA, et al., 2015]. Pre-washed bagged nonstarchy vegetables although technically 'processed,' are not what I'm talking about when I suggest staying away from processed foods. The processed foods that should be avoided are made in a factory from grains, sugar, and vegetable oils and have high-glycemic indices and loads. No existing exogenous insulin can fully compensate for the rapid rise in post-meal blood sugar that results. That said, there are some whole, unprocessed foods, that raise blood glucose significantly, e.g. potatoes and most fruits, and may need to be minimized or avoided completely. With time and more familiarity with the carbohydrate content and ingredients of some minimally-processed foods, you can experiment with using some for your convenience. Cheese is a processed food, but there are many different types of cheese with different ingredients such that some are very healthful, e.g., aged cheddar cheese, while others, e.g., Cheese Whiz (contains canola oil and maltodextrin), are not.

Table 4.1 — Glycemic Index of Foods

Low Glycemic Index Foods Acceptable in a LCD	Glycemic Index	High Glycemic Index Foods To Avoid in a LCD	Glycemic Index
Asparagus	10	Green Peas	48
Broccoli	10	Spaghetti, white	50
Bell Pepper	10	Carrots, cooked	50
Cabbage	10	Kiwi fruit	52
Cauliflower	10	Sweet corn	52
Green Beans	10	Specialty grain bread	53

Lettuce	10	Couscous	65
Mushrooms	10	White rice, boiled	73
Onions	10	White wheat bread	75
Tomato	15	Roasted Potato	85
Carrots, raw	16	White rice, instant	90
Grapefruit	25	Dextrose (glucose)	100

A Well-Formulated Low-Carbohydrate Diet

Stephen Phinney, MD, PhD and Jeff Volek, RD, PhD coined the terms 'well-formulated low-carbohydrate diet' as well as 'nutritional ketosis' and 'keto-adaptation' [Volek, JS, et al., 2011a]. A well-formulated LCD simply means that it is properly constructed to be sustainable long-term without adverse side-effects. A list of attributes of a well-formulated LCD/VLCD include the following:

1. For those with T1D, a LCD/VLCD facilitates normalization of or improvement in blood sugars and reduces glycemic variability, hypoglycemic episodes, and TDID. Embarking on a LCD without appropriate reduction in insulin doses can result in hypoglycemia. Ongoing medical supervision is recommended to help you adjust medications and insulin doses.
2. Supports lean body mass (muscle), sheds body fat, and adequately fuels exercise and sports performance.
3. Includes adequate intake of electrolytes (sodium and potassium), minerals (magnesium), and water to prevent dizziness, fatigue, headache, constipation, and other symptoms of dehydration, mineral and/or electrolyte imbalance.

4. Fat, including saturated fat, naturally found in meat, fish, poultry, eggs, butter, cheese, nuts, seeds, olives, coconuts, avocados, etc. provide most of one's energy needs and should not be avoided due to false concerns about the development of CVD.
5. A LCD is composed predominantly of nutritious whole foods with minimal processed foods, even those specifically designed for a LCD, VLCD, or 'keto' diet.
6. Very low-calorie diets and fasting beyond 24 hours could increase the risk of DKA and should be avoided in those with T1D.
7. A LCD avoids all vegetable/seed oils. The polyunsaturated fatty acids (PUFA) in vegetable oils lead to chronic systemic inflammation and likely contribute to the causation of several modern chronic diseases [DiNicolantonio, JJ, et al., 2018, Teicholz, N, 2010]. These oils are used as ingredients in processed foods and restaurants fry foods in vegetable oils. Some LCD foods, e.g., nuts & seeds, are roasted dry or in oil which can damage the PUFA in the nuts/seeds and in the vegetable oil. I prefer to eat them raw and avoid oil-fried, oil-roasted, and dry-roasted nuts & seeds just to be sure. Vegetable oils to be avoided include safflower seed, grape seed, sunflower seed, silybum seed, hemp seed, wheat germ, corn, pumpkin seed, cottonseed, soybean, sesame seed, rice bran, peanut (a legume, not a nut), and canola (rapeseed).
8. Although the LCD/VLCD is a major part of improving blood sugar control, the other strategies discussed in this book should be implemented as well to normalize blood sugars.

You may also want to read *Ten Defining Characteristics of a Well-Formulated Ketogenic Diet* at https://blog.virtahealth.com/well-formulated-ketogenic-diet/. Some who start a well-formulated LCD may experience temporary symptoms of fatigue and reduced athletic performance while their body is keto-adapting. Most who experience unwanted 'side-effects' do so as a result of a poorly-formulated LCD. This is often the basis for myths about the 'harms of a LCD.' Thus, the difference between a well- and poorly-formulated LCD is paying attention to the details and being compliant with the instructions. I spent several weeks reading about the details of a VLCD before beginning and experienced no adverse effects. Proper formulation of your LCD can make the difference between success and failure in most cases. When success has not been achieved, many will blame the diet for being intolerable or ineffective, when it was their own improper formulation of the LCD that was the real culprit. Some of the adverse 'side-effects' of a poorly-formulated LCD include constipation, muscle cramps, and the 'Atkins flu' which includes fatigue, dizziness, achiness, and headaches.

The most common mistakes are:
1. Not drinking enough water → 'Atkins flu,' fatigue, dizziness, headaches, and constipation.
2. Not adding enough salt to food → 'Atkins flu.'
3. Eating too much dietary fat or food in general → gain unwanted body fat or unable to lose body fat.
4. Exceeding one's daily carbohydrate goal → less than optimal blood sugars or unable to achieve nutritional ketosis when one's goal is to do so.
5. Specifically avoiding dietary fat or not eating enough food → losing unwanted bodyweight.
6. Sedentary lifestyle → constipation.
7. Insufficient magnesium intake or excessive exercise → muscle cramps (helped by increasing green leafy vegetables, taking magnesium chloride or Slow Mag, or reducing exercise).

One physiologic explanation for the consequences of not consuming enough salt and water is that the kidneys respond to reduced insulin levels by increasing the excretion of both salt and water. As long as you continue the LCD, the kidneys will continue to excrete more salt and water than before starting the LCD. Thus, part of your new lifestyle will be to increase salt and water intake henceforth. It is analogous to moving to a dessert environment. If you do not continue drinking additional water everyday, you will become dehydrated. Those with medical conditions including high blood pressure, congestive heart failure, advanced kidney or liver disease, or other fluid-retaining conditions should consult with their physician for advice on the appropriate salt and water intake for their condition.

The Low-Carbohydrate Diet

A LCD allows a larger selection and/or quantity of low-glycemic index foods with 51–100 grams of total dietary carbohydrate/day making it more sustainable in the long-term as long as you can achieve your glycemic goals. A LCD can produce marked improvements in glycemic control. A clinical audit [Nielsen, JV, et al., 2012] of 48 T1D patients who were instructed to follow a 75-gram/day LCD and followed for four years found that after one year, the average mealtime bolus insulin dosage of 36 of the 48 patients decreased from 23 IU to 13 IU and the basal insulin dosage decreased from 19.6 IU to 18.6 IU. The TDID decreased by 26% from 42.6 IU to 31.6 IU. Symptomatic hypoglycemia decreased by 82% after one year. The 18 patients who adhered to the LCD for four years experienced a sustained reduction in HbA1c from 7.8% to 6.0% (a 23% decrease).

The Very Low-Carbohydrate Diet

A VLCD allows up to 50 grams of total dietary carbohydrate/day to achieve your glycemic goals and typically results in nutritional ketosis. Nutritional ketosis is a normal physiologic reaction to dietary carbohydrate restriction whereupon insulin levels decline and glucagon levels increase signaling the liver to make ketones and glucose to fuel organs, particularly the brain, that are less able to use fatty acids (see Chapter 13). The exact amount of total dietary carbohydrate/day you choose is a balance between your ability to reach your glycemic goals and your ability to construct a VLCD that you can enjoy day-in and day-out for the rest of your life. Use of a VLCD may translate to better control of blood sugars and lower insulin doses compared to a LCD. The foods eaten on a VLCD are essentially the same as for the LCD, but a VLCD does restrict the amount of some low-carbohydrate foods including fruit, nonstarchy vegetables, nuts & seeds, and some dairy products. For most individuals, this reduction will not interfere with obtaining enough of the essential vitamins and minerals. A VLCD is also particularly helpful for those with 'double diabetes.' Double diabetes is a term coined in 2001 to describe the combination of T1D and features of T2D including insulin resistance, obesity, metabolic syndrome, chronic inflammation, and higher insulin doses [Dandona, P, et al., 2005]. Those with double diabetes may require a 20 gram/day carbohydrate restriction to resolve insulin resistance and improve body composition. While restricting and/or eliminating foods one enjoys may seem undesirable when first beginning a VLCD, once the transition is made, most find they feel satisfied with each and every meal, i.e., being neither hungry, nor wanting for more, and that matters more than eating any particular food.

A VLCD can markedly improve glycemic control in those with T1D. In this online survey [Lennerz, BS, et al., 2018], 316 children and adults were "… recruited from TypeOneGrit, an online Facebook community for people with T1D who follow a VLCD and diabetes management method as recommended in the book, *Dr Bernstein's Diabetes Solution*. This method comprises a VLCD with weight-based carbohydrate prescription of up to 30 g per day derived from fibrous vegetables and nuts with a low glycemic index. High-protein foods with associated fat are substituted for carbohydrates and adjusted on the basis of outcomes, including glycemic control and weight. Participants adhere to a structured meal plan and adjust bolus insulin empirically according to postprandial glycemia. Basal insulin is adjusted according to fasting glycemia." The survey respondents had been on the VLCD for a mean duration of 2.2 years and the mean carbohydrate intake was 36 g/day. The mean HbA1c decreased from 7.12% to 5.67% (−1.45% or a 20% reduction), mean blood glucose was 106 mg/dl (5.9 mM), SDBG was 36 mg/dl (2.0 mM) with only 7 (2%) respondents reporting diabetes-related hospitalizations in the past year, including 4 (1%) for ketoacidosis and 2 (1%) for hypoglycemia. This is the lowest published HbA1c that I have seen in persons with T1D. Although the survey respondents were asked under what circumstances they would measure ketones and the ketone levels that would concern them, they were not asked to report their ketone results, and thus, they were not reported in the study. The survey is available at https://osf.io/d6wrj/.

The Ketogenic Ratio

In 1921, Shaffer proposed the ketogenic ratio (KR): the ratio of the sum of ketogenic factors to the sum of antiketogenic factors in the diet of man [Shaffer, PA, 1921]. In 1980, Withrow [Withrow, CD, 1980] modified the equation for the KR as follows: $KR = (0.9\,F + 0.46\,P) \div (C + 0.58\,P + 0.1\,F)$

where F is grams of dietary fat, P is grams of dietary protein, and C is grams of dietary carbohydrate. From the equation, we can see that carbohydrate is 100% antiketogenic, fat is 90% ketogenic and 10% antiketogenic, and protein is 46% ketogenic and 58% antiketogenic. Therefore, the major determinants of a diet's ability to produce ketosis are its carbohydrate and fat content, whereas its protein content has only a minor effect on ketosis. The KR can range from 0 (glucose) to 9 (pure fat). Using Withrow's equation, this study [Zilberter, T, et al., 2018] found that a diet with a KR ≥ 1.7 likely results in nutritional ketosis in humans. They also enumerated some of the potential advantages of a ketogenic VLCD compared to a LFHCD: "The metabolic effects of dietary fat on energy homeostasis differs from the effects of carbohydrates in two key features. One is the ability to store energy in depots — fat is exceptionally good at it, but carbohydrates are limited in this ability. The other is the ability to increase the drive to consume energy. Carbohydrates have a characteristic ability to elicit positive reward and thus addiction while significant carbohydrate restriction in VLCD caused not only energy intake decrease, but also energy expenditure increase in both resting and active states. In spite of these non-homeostatic features, these mechanisms are evolutionarily appropriate in wild nature, but as soon as the living conditions change the hard-wired pursuit to maximize the energy store becomes a metabolic trap, resulting in non-homeostatic overconsumption and all the negative metabolic consequences it causes."

How to Design and Begin Your Low-Carbohydrate Diet

Table 4.2 contains the type of foods you should eat and avoid on a LCD. Having everyone in the family adopt the same LCD makes following and complying with the diet easier for the T1D especially if no excluded foods are available in the house. Other family members will often notice unexpected benefits as well. Knowing which foods to avoid on a LCD is very important, and fortunately, the list is rather short: any food or drink containing more than a tiny amount of sugar (natural or added sugar), starch, vegetable oil, and alcohol.

Table 4.2 — Foods to Eat and Avoid on a Low-Carbohydrate Diet

Eat These Foods	Avoid These Foods Entirely
Meat & Eggs: Beef, pork, lamb, game, poultry, and eggs: all types. There is no need to remove the fat or skin from meat or poultry. If having difficulty losing weight, choose leaner meats.	Sugar: Soft drinks, candy, fruit juice, sports drinks, chocolate, cakes, buns, pastries, ice cream and breakfast cereals. Artificial sweeteners can cause some to have sugar cravings.
Fish and seafood: All kinds, but preferably fatty fish such as salmon, mackerel, or herring which are high in omega-3 fatty acids, EPA and DHA.	Starches: All grains, bread, pasta, rice, cereal, potatoes, corn-based products, French fries, potato chips, porridge, oatmeal, root vegetables.
Fats: Tallow, lard, suet, cheese, butter, ghee, cream, coconut cream, avocado oil, coconut oil, macadamia oil, unadulterated olive oil, MCT oil.	Vegetable oils, shortenings, & margarine
Dairy: All dairy should be full-fat, with attention to total carb content, aged-cheese, butter, ghee, cream, and whole milk yogurt are low-carb.	Dairy: Avoid reduced-fat dairy products, milk, Kifer, yogurt with added fruit or sugar.
Vegetables & Fruits: All kinds of nonstarchy vegetables: cabbage, collard greens, kale, green beans, broccoli, asparagus, yellow squash, zucchini, cucumber, lettuce, olives, avocado, limited amounts of raspberries, blackberries and strawberries, melon, peach, lemon, grapefruit.	Fruits: most fruit contains lots of sugar and fructose. Avoid all dried fruits and most fresh fruits except as listed on the left, in limited quantities.

Nuts & Seeds: Pecans, walnuts, macadamia, pistachios, almonds, hazelnuts, Brazil nuts, best when eaten raw (my bias), rather than dry or oil roasted. Limit amounts for weight loss.	Alcohol: all types should be avoided in those with diabetes (it can cause hypoglycemia). Alcohol is a liver toxin and contains calories absent of any nutrients. Alcohol slows weight loss.
Drinks: Unsweetened water, tea & coffee, using herbal tea after dinner, rather than caffeinated tea & coffee, helps many to fall asleep.	Drinks: Alcohol, sweetened drinks, fruit juice, and diet drinks with artificial sweeteners should be avoided.

Tables 4.3–4.8 list the grams of protein, carbohydrate, and fat per 100 g of various foods as well as the KR for those who decide to follow a ketogenic VLCD is also included. As mentioned, diets with a KR ≥ 1.7 typically result in nutritional ketosis. Common foods on a LCD include beef, lamb, pork, fish, poultry, eggs (Table 4.3), dairy products (Table 4.4), nonstarchy vegetables (Table 4.5), nuts & seeds (Table 4.6), lower-sugar fruits (Table 4.7), and fats and oils (Table 4.8).

Table 4.3 — Low-Carbohydrate Meat, Fish, Poultry, Eggs

Food	Protein	Carbs	Fat	KR
Lamb	22.5	0.0	20.0	1.88
Chicken Eggs	12.6	1.1	10.6	1.62
Ground Beef, 80% lean	25.3	0.0	16.2	1.61
Pork	27.0	0.0	15.2	1.52
Chicken, thigh	28.2	0.0	13.2	1.41
Salmon	25.4	0.0	8.1	1.22
Chicken, breast	30.9	0.0	4.5	0.99
Tilapia	26.2	0.0	2.7	0.94

| Turkey, breast | 30.1 | 0.0 | 2.1 | 0.89 |

Table 4.4 — Dairy Products

Food	Protein	Carbs	Fat	KR
Ghee	0.3	0.0	99.5	8.86
Butter	0.9	0.1	81.1	8.41
Cream, heavy whipping	2.8	2.7	36.1	4.26
Sour Cream	2.4	4.6	19.4	2.34
Cream cheese	5.3	4.7	20.7	2.14
Cheddar cheese, sharp	23.8	4.8	33.3	1.87
Yogurt, Plain, 4% Whole Milk	3.5	4.7	3.3	0.65
Kefir, Low-fat	3.5	4.7	3.3	0.65
Milk, Whole	3.2	4.8	3.3	0.64

Table 4.5 — Non-Starchy Vegetables

Food	Protein	Carbs	Fat	KR
Zucchini, cooked	1.1	2.7	0.4	0.26
Collard Greens, cooked	2.7	5.7	0.7	0.26
Kale, raw	4.3	8.8	0.9	0.24
Romaine lettuce	1.2	3.3	0.3	0.20
Broccoli, cooked	2.4	7.2	0.4	0.17
Summer squash, cooked	0.9	4.3	0.3	0.14
Cabbage, green, cooked	1.3	5.5	0.1	0.11

Table 4.6 — Nuts & Seeds

Food	Protein	Carbs	Fat	KR
Macadamia nuts	7.9	13.8	75.8	2.77
Pecans	9.2	13.9	72.0	2.61
Brazil nuts	14.3	11.7	67.1	2.51
Almonds	15.2	13.7	65.2	2.26
Walnuts	15.2	13.7	65.2	2.26
Hazelnuts	15.0	16.7	60.8	1.96
Pumpkin seeds	29.8	14.7	49.1	1.57
Sunflower seeds	20.8	20.0	51.5	1.50
Pistachios	20.2	27.2	45.3	1.15
Cashews	18.2	30.2	43.9	1.06

Table 4.7 — Lower Sugar Fruits

Food	Protein	Carbs	Fat	KR
Ripe Olives	0.8	6.0	10.9	1.35
Avocado, black skin	2.0	8.6	15.4	1.31
Starfruit	1.0	6.7	0.3	0.10
Raspberry	1.2	11.9	0.7	0.09
Lemon	1.1	9.3	0.3	0.08
Strawberry	0.7	7.7	0.3	0.07
Watermelon	0.6	7.6	0.2	0.06
Lemon juice	0.4	6.9	0.2	0.05
Grapefruit	0.8	10.7	0.1	0.04

| Blueberry | 0.7 | 14.5 | 0.3 | 0.04 |

Table 4.8 — Fats & Oils

Food	Protein	Carbs	Fat	KR
Lard, suet, tallow, or duck fat	0.0	0.0	100.0	9.00
Olive, Coconut, or MCT oil	0.0	0.0	100.0	9.00

Formulating Meals with cronometer.com and dietdoctor.com

The easiest method to normalize blood sugars and improve body composition is to quantitate the number of grams of protein, carbohydrate, and fat in each meal using the free web application: cronometer.com. In a few minutes, most can learn how to navigate this free application. It will calculate the quantities of macronutrients (protein, carbohydrate, and fat) and micronutrients (vitamins and minerals) of any food, meal, or an entire day of eating using any portions you specify. It presents a calendar allowing you to log foods eaten daily, but I don't use it for that purpose. Instead, I use the application to design each of my three daily meals. Using the app ensures my meals meet my daily macronutrient targets for a VLCD and reach 100% of the recommended daily allowance (RDA) for all the micronutrients. As explained in Chapter 3, no database is perfectly accurate, but this is not a problem because once a meal is formulated, it is repeated until you need a change. **In other words, day-to-day consistency of meals is more important than an exact amount of any particular nutrient in terms of blood glucose control.** This is because BID should be determined based on the blood glucose response to the BID on previous days for the same meal at the same time of day. I found through experience that trying to base insulin doses on grams of carbohydrate or protein is not helpful due to the inaccuracies of these nutrient databases and the fact that one's response to bolus insulin is a function of multiple other factors in addition to meal macronutrients. Thus, basing BID on the blood glucose response to BID on previous day(s) takes all of the pertinent factors, i.e., macronutrients, exercise, sleep, etc., into account. I suggest changing meals no more frequently than once a week which facilitates achieving normal blood sugars. Getting as many of your micronutrients from food as possible is preferable, but using a vitamin or mineral supplement is acceptable as well. When I desire a change in meals, I simply go back to cronometer.com and design a new meal. Another useful website is dietdoctor.com. This website has easy-to-understand low-carb information in written and video formats with delicious recipes that make the low-carb lifestyle enjoyable and sustainable. I have included only one recipe in this book because dietdoctor.com has so many well-formulated low-carb recipes ready for you to use. There are numerous other websites and books with low-carb recipes as well. It is important that you enter any recipe you plan to use into cronometer.com for the purposes described in this chapter.

The first step in the design process is to determine your goal intake of total daily carbohydrate, protein, and fat (in grams). Quantifying all the dietary macronutrients is the best method to ensure that, 1) dietary carbohydrate is adequately restricted, 2) dietary protein is high enough to maintain or build lean muscle mass, 3) dietary fat is set to maintain or improve your body composition, and 4) blood sugars can be normalized with predictable BID. Each macronutrient has different insulin requirements (carbohydrates > protein > fat), but because these requirements are not known, the most effective strategy is to simply keep all of the macronutrients in each meal constant from day to day. The easiest way to accomplish this is to eat the same meal, at any given time of day, everyday. Breakfast, lunch, and dinner can be different, of course, since each meal will have a different BID. You don't need to design every aspect of your LCD perfectly from day one. We all need to start somewhere and then adjust it over time to meet our goals or to adjust for changes in our bodies, preferences, circumstances, etc. Since beginning my VLCD in 2012, I have made numerous small changes in the number meals eaten per day, i.e., 2, 3, and 4 meals/day, or the choice of foods to add variety or to test for food intolerances or to add micronutrients or to change my bodyweight to a different weight class for olympic weightlifting. Each dietary change I make is small and I wait 1–3 weeks between changes to allow my blood sugar and insulin doses to stabilize.

Why Micronutrients Matter

I suggest designing your LCD/VLCD so that it supplies as close to 100% of the RDA of vitamins and minerals as possible while also taking note of the precautions listed above regarding salt, sodium, potassium, and magnesium intake for those with medical conditions. There are three additional essential micronutrients, chromium, molybdenum, and vitamin K2, that are not shown on cronometer.com. Good sources of chromium include eggs, cheese, broccoli, tomatoes, green beans, and romaine lettuce. Good sources of molybdenum include sesame seeds, walnuts, almonds, and eggs. Good sources of vitamin K2 include pork, eggs, cheese, fermented foods, and butter. Vitamin C is plentiful in fruit, but since fruit is limited in a LCD, the second most abundant food source is vegetables. However, vitamin C is destroyed by overcooking vegetables or prolonged storage. Vegetables high in vitamin C include bell peppers, tomatoes, and broccoli which can be eaten raw or lightly steamed. Supplements can be utilized as well.

In addition to developing the Ames test to detect whether a given chemical can cause mutations in the DNA of a test organism, Dr. Bruce Ames, PhD also proposed the 'triage theory' of micronutrients [Ames, BN, 2006]. He points out that Americans are not getting adequate amounts of certain micronutrients that play a critical role in DNA repair. When these micronutrients are in short supply, the body triages the micronutrients it does get to their most essential roles, preventing disease and death in the short-term, but leaves other processes, e.g., repairing DNA mutations, without the necessary cofactors to function properly. Thus mild micronutrient deficiencies occurring over many years can manifest as cancer because DNA mutations were unable to be repaired. This review article discusses the levels of micronutrient intake needed to protect the integrity of DNA further emphasizing the importance of consuming a diet that is sufficient in micronutrients for long-term health [Fenech, MF, 2010]. This website's nutrient search tool is helpful to find foods that are high in a particular micronutrient, https://nutritiondata.self.com/tools/nutrient-search, and is also free. You can use Table 4.9, cronometer.com, https://www.ncbi.nlm.nih.gov/books/NBK56068/table/summarytables.t2/?report=objectonly, for vitamin recommended daily intake (RDI), and https://www.ncbi.nlm.nih.gov/books/NBK545442/table/appJ_tab3/?report=objectonly, for mineral RDIs, as checklists to make sure you get all of your essential nutrients.

Table 4.9 — The 40 Essential Nutrients

Biotin	Iron	Niacin B3	Threonine
Calcium	Isoleucine	Pantothenate B5	Tryptophan
Chloride	Leucine	Phenylalanine	Valine
Choline	Linoleic Acid	Phosphorus	Vitamin A

Chromium	Linolenic Acid	Potassium	Vitamin B12
Cobalt	Lysine	Pyridoxine B6	Vitamin C
Copper	Magnesium	Riboflavin B2	Vitamin D
Folate B9	Manganese	Selenium	Vitamin E
Histidine	Methionine	Sodium	Vitamin K
Iodide	Molybdenum	Thiamine B1	Zinc

Select Your Dietary Carbohydrate Intake

When designing your well-formulated LCD, you first have to select a dietary carbohydrate goal to aim for using the information given above. If you haven't yet decided whether to start with a LCD or a VLCD, you can start designing meals you like, emphasizing low-glycemic load foods, and just see where the daily carbohydrate intake comes out. Then, gradually adjust it over several weeks, if needed, to a carbohydrate intake that results in a diet you enjoy and is bringing you closer to accomplishing your glycemic and bodyweight goals. A slower rate of reduction in carbohydrates can allow for smaller and more gradual reductions in insulin doses. The pace of change is really up to you.

Starch and Sugars Hidden in Processed Foods

The most common sugars in the diet include sucrose (from sugar cane and beets), glucose (from starches), fructose (from fruit, honey, agave, and high-fructose corn syrup), and lactose (from milk). Sucrose, or table sugar, breaks down to glucose and fructose in equal proportions upon digestion. Starches include grains (wheat, corn, rice, and quinoa), starchy vegetables (potatoes), and legumes (black, kidney, and lima beans, peanuts, chickpeas, green, snow, snap, split, and black-eyed peas, and lentils) which break down to glucose upon digestion. Glucose is the sugar in the blood that we measure when checking our blood sugar. It should be no surprise that sugars and starches raise blood sugar so dramatically!

There are at least 56 different names for sugar used on processed food ingredient labels as shown in Table 4.10. This is on purpose, of course, because the food industry knows their customers are trying to limit their consumption of sugar. They use these 56 different names in the hopes you will not recognize one or more of them as sugar. This also allows them to place the name of the sugar in the later portion of the ingredient list which is required to be listed from most abundant to least abundant. If they named all sugars as 'sugar,' then it would appear near the front of the list and be easily recognized. **More than 70% of processed foods have added sugar** [Ng, SW, et al., 2012]. Many of these processed foods are savory, rather than sweet, and most people would not even suspect that they contain added sugar. Thus, many people do not even look at the label to see if it contains sugar or how much it contains. I have seen ingredient labels with four different names for sugar. The food industry knows that by adding sugar to its processed foods, their customers will eat more of the food and be more likely to purchase it again. Bottomline, if you do eat some processed foods, use the total carbohydrate (grams) on the Nutrition Facts label (or in <u>cronometer.com</u>) when designing a meal. Note that the total carbohydrate is 'per serving,' not the entire container. For example, if the label says, 18 grams total carbohydrate per serving, and contains 3 servings, the entire container has 54 grams of total carbohydrate.

Table 4.10 — Fifty-Six Names for Sugar

| Agave Nectar/Syrup | Galactose |

Master Type 1 Diabetes

Barley malt	Glucose
Beet sugar	Glucose syrup solids
Blackstrap molasses	Golden sugar
Brown rice syrup	Golden syrup
Brown sugar	Grape sugar
Buttered sugar/buttercream	High-Fructose Corn Syrup (HFCS)
Cane juice crystals	Honey
Cane sugar	Icing sugar
Caramel	Invert sugar
Carob syrup	Lactose
Castor sugar	Malt syrup
Coconut sugar	Maltodextrin
Confectioner's sugar	Maltose
Corn syrup	Maple syrup
Corn syrup solids	Molasses
Crystalline fructose	Muscovado sugar
Date sugar	Panela sugar
Demerara sugar	Raw sugar
Dextrin	Refiner's syrup
Dextrose	Rice syrup
Diastatic malt	Sorghum syrup
Ethyl maltol	Sucanat
Evaporated cane juice	Sucrose

Florida crystals	Sugar (granulated or table)
Fructose	Treacle
Fruit juice	Turbinado sugar
Fruit juice concentrate	Yellow sugar

Foods with significant amounts of refined carbohydrates and sugar can be addictive and you may miss eating them after starting your LCD. This is understandable, but within ≈ 6 weeks of abstention, the desire to consume them will dissipate. Food industry scientists purposefully design foods to 1) send reinforcing signals to the brain, 2) create addiction, and 3) maximize food consumption. Howard Moskowitz, a food industry consultant, coined the term 'bliss point' to describe the optimal combination of salt, sugar, and fat in processed foods that would maximize food consumption in test subjects. He helped develop many food products like spaghetti sauce and soft drinks using his 'bliss point' method [Moss, M, 2013]. Additionally, do not think that artificial sweeteners are a solution to sugar addiction: quite the opposite. Artificial sweeteners can simply extend your sugar addiction and make resisting trigger foods more difficult [Yang, Q, 2010].

Calculate Goal Bodyweight and Daily Caloric Requirement

Quantitating macronutrient intake is an effective strategy to normalize blood sugars and improve body composition in those with T1D. I will take you through the steps needed to accomplish this. We will need a goal bodyweight to calculate caloric and protein intake. If you are satisfied with your current bodyweight, you will use it as your goal bodyweight and calculate your current caloric intake with cronometer.com by entering everything you typically eat in a day. If you desire to lose body fat, you can choose a goal bodyweight or use this free calculator, https://www.calculator.net/ideal-weight-calculator.html, to help you determine your goal bodyweight and then use https://www.calculator.net/calorie-calculator.html, to calculate your daily caloric requirement.

Calculate Daily Dietary Protein and Fat Intake

Now that you have chosen your goal bodyweight and daily caloric and carbohydrate intake, you need to choose your daily protein intake and calculate your fat intake. Dietary protein should be quantified because of its essential role in growth and maintenance of lean muscle mass as well as its effect on blood sugar. Most Americans are not eating enough dietary protein and combined with their lack of exercise results in sarcopenia (small and weak muscles) and osteoporosis (thin bones that fracture more easily). Dietary protein intake, based on your goal bodyweight, is chosen within the ranges shown in Table 4.11. These levels of protein intake are based on the 95% confidence interval of protein intake from this meta-analysis [Morton, RW, et al., 2018]. Determining dietary protein intake is an inexact science and my bias, if one must err on one side or the other, is in the direction of 'more-than-enough.' The ranges in Table 4.11 are designed to give you flexibility in determining whether you prefer a somewhat lower or somewhat higher protein intake. I prefer a higher protein intake to support my athletic pursuits and muscle mass as I age. A higher protein intake also helps to suppress appetite and preserve lean muscle mass when losing body fat [Longland, TM, et al., 2016, Murphy, CH, et al., 2015]. Those who are less concerned about retaining muscle mass and want to maximize ketone levels may prefer a lower protein intake. In young persons, each meal should contain ≥ 25 grams of protein and ≥ 2 grams of leucine to maximize muscle protein synthesis (MPS).

Older persons should aim for 30–40 grams of protein and 2.5–3 grams of leucine at each meal, due to age-related anabolic resistance [Wall, BT, et al., 2015]. Resistance exercise is an effective method for preserving lean muscle mass especially when losing body fat [Layman, DK, et al., 2005]. You might ask, 'Is it possible to eat too much protein?' In short, 'For those with normal kidney function, no.' Protein intakes above 2.2 grams/kg BW/day during a 2-year study period demonstrated no deleterious effects in those with normal kidney function [Antonio, J, et al., 2018].

Table 4.11 — Suggested Daily Protein Intake

Physical Activity Level	Sedentary, Light, or Moderate Activity	Moderate, Very Active, or Losing Body Fat	Extra Active or Gaining Muscle
Protein Intake (g/kg goal BW/day	1.2–1.6	1.7–2.2	≥ 2.3
Minimum Protein Intake Per Meal (g)	30	40	50

Note: Persons with advanced chronic kidney disease (CKD), stages 3b–5 may benefit from protein restriction, 0.6–0.8 grams/kg bodyweight/day, so you should consult with your nephrologist before making any changes to your diet.

Once goal carbohydrate and protein grams and total caloric intake has been determined, fat grams are calculated next:
1. Calculated carbohydrate calories = Goal daily carbohydrate grams × 4 kcal/g.
2. Choose a goal daily protein intake ≥ 1.2 g/kg/day from Table 4.11 above.

3. Goal daily protein intake (grams) = goal or 'ideal' or bodyweight (kg) × goal daily protein intake (in g/kg/day). To convert lb. to kg, divide by 2.2 lb./kg.
4. Calculated protein calories = Goal daily protein grams × 4 kcal/g.
5. Calculated fat calories = Goal total daily calories − Calculated protein calories − Goal carbohydrate calories.
6. Calculated fat grams = Calculated fat calories ÷ 9 kcal/g.

Here's an example, using my entry data:
My caloric intake using cronometer.com is 2,722 kcal/day.
I have chosen 39 grams/day carbohydrate intake.
From Table 4.11 above, I chose a goal daily protein intake of 2.3 g/kg/day.

The calculations are as follows:
Calculated carbohydrate calories = 39 × 4 kcal/g = 156 kcal/day.
Convert bodyweight from pounds (lb.) to kilograms (kg): 160 lb. ÷ 2.2 lb./kg = 72.7 kg
Goal daily protein intake (g/day) = 72.7 kg × 2.3 g/kg/day = 167 g/day.
Calculated protein calories = 167 g/day × 4 kcal/g = 669 kcal/day.
Calculated fat calories = 2,722 kcal/day − 156 kcal/day − 669 kcal/day = 1,897 kcal/day.
Calculated fat grams = 1,897 kcal/day ÷ 9 kcal/g = 211 grams/day.

Using cronometer.com, you can design 1, 2, 3, or 4 meals/day by dividing the calculated grams/day of carbohydrate, protein, and fat calculated above by 1, 2, 3, or 4, respectively. I chose to eat three meals/day, so I divided the grams above by 3.
Goal carbohydrate grams = 39 grams/day ÷ 3 meals/day = 13 grams/meal.

Calculated protein grams = 167 grams/day ÷ 3 meals/day = 56 grams/meal.
Calculated fat grams = 211 grams/day ÷ 3 meals/day = 70 grams/meal.

Then, design your meals close to these macronutrients. Macronutrients in each meal can be different as long as all the meals add up to your daily total and they don't vary from day to day. In terms of blood sugar control, the fewer different meals you rotate through at any given meal, the better. You can use your own judgement as to how often you change them. Sticking with the same meal for a least one week seems to work best in terms of achieving normal blood sugars. Preparing meals on the weekend for the week and storing them in separate containers in the refrigerator or freezer is an easy way to have standardized meals for home, school, or work.

How Many Meals Per Day?

After experimenting with 2, 3, and 4 meals/day, I found eating 3 meals/day conforms to social norms, preserves lean muscle mass, and facilitates controlling blood sugars with moderate-sized BID. It is a bit awkward to eat meals out-of-sync with family and coworkers. Eating 4 meals/day provides more potential opportunities to maximize MPS and the ability to give smaller insulin doses with each meal. If the 4th meal is before bedtime, it shouldn't interfere with other family members' norms. I tested this strategy in 2019 for several months. I ate the 4th meal at 10 PM just before going to bed. My blood sugars were normal, but no better than with three meals/day. I couldn't detect any difference in muscle mass or strength and it did take extra time to cook, eat, and clean-up, so I decided on 3 meals/day. As mentioned in Chapter 2, I ate only breakfast and dinner for 13 years just to reduce the risk of hypoglycemia while at work.

Had I known about the LCD and the other strategies discussed in this book, I could have eaten lunch while at work. Although I have never tried it, eating one meal/day is possible and might help some to lose body fat. It would require a larger BID. If I did try it, I would eat my one meal at breakfast to control the dawn phenomenon, i.e., the early morning cortisol release from the adrenal glands [Porcellati, F, et al., 2013]. Skipping breakfast may work well for some, but others may experience an increase in blood sugar after waking up due to the dawn phenomenon. To compensate for the dawn phenomenon, a morning correction insulin dose can be taken or alternatively, the correction dose can be incorporated into the breakfast mealtime bolus dose. Fasting beyond 24 hours is not prudent for those with T1D. Each day you go without food your TDID will decline. Because there is a lag in the blood glucose response to changes in basal insulin dosage compared to bolus insulin, it will be difficult to keep blood sugars normal during a prolonged fast. More importantly, the lower TDID could increase the risk of developing DKA or euglycemic DKA (euDKA) since exogenous insulin does not regulate glucagon levels and liver glucose and ketone production as precisely as endogenous β-cell insulin. Euglycemic DKA is DKA with a blood sugar less than 200 mg/dl (11.1 mM). Another disadvantage to prolonged fasting is muscle protein loss since it is used as a substrate for gluconeogenesis by the liver and kidneys to make glucose (gluconeogenesis) [see Fig. 1, Owen, OE, 2005]. As mentioned previously, there are numerous benefits to retaining muscle mass as we age from the perspective of strength as well as metabolic health since muscle is the largest consumer of glucose in our bodies. The potential benefits of fasting beyond 24 hours are not worth the risks in those with T1D.

Adjusting Dietary Fat Intake to Lose Body Fat

For those who need to lose body fat, choosing a LCD/VLCD helps to control of hunger to create the necessary caloric deficit. Because a LCD is already low in dietary carbohydrate and dietary protein is essentially fixed to maintain lean body mass, dietary fat is the remaining macronutrient that can be reduced. The simplest strategy is to reduce dietary fat in 22 gram/day (or 200 kcal/day) steps. Progress can be tracked with weekly waist circumference, bodyweight measurements upon arising from bed in the morning, and your appearance in a mirror. Remember that bodyweight is a combination of lean body mass (primarily bone, muscle, and organs) and fat mass. If you are losing body fat and gaining lean body mass at the same time (both desirable), your bodyweight could remain unchanged. Thus waist circumference and body appearance can be more reliable measures of body fat mass than a scale. A waist-to-height ratio of < 0.5 correlates with metabolic health and is a useful goal to aim for [Ferreira-Hermosillo, A, et al., 2014]. Body composition testing with a DEXA scan, BOD POD®, calipers, or hydrostatic underwater weighing is another option to track body fat loss. The downsides of using these testing methods include inaccuracy, cost, and radiation exposure in the case of DEXA scanning. If you don't seem to be heading in the right direction after several weeks, your dietary fat intake can be reduced by another 22 grams/day as long as you are not having any symptoms of insufficient caloric intake which include hunger, increasing thoughts of food, desire to eat more, fatigue, lack of desire for physical activity, constipation, and feeling cold, irritable, or anxious. Physical activity, either aerobic or resistance training, or both, modestly assists in losing body fat primarily by increasing muscle mass and caloric expenditure [Swift, DL, et al., 2014], and helps those with T1D by increasing muscular glucose consumption and improving insulin sensitivity with reduced insulin doses. Resistance exercise is an effective method for building and preserving lean muscle mass especially when losing body fat [Layman, DK, et al., 2005].

Meal Design, Timing & Muscle Protein Synthesis

Note above that I divided my total daily protein intake by three so that each meal has the same protein intake. Most Americans typically consume their daily protein unevenly across the day with the least at breakfast and the most at dinner. This study showed that consuming protein evenly across all meals resulted in a 25% increase in MPS [Mamerow, MM, et al., 2014]. A similar study [Yasuda, J, et al., 2020] found greater lean muscle mass (LMM) gain (+2.5 kg LMM vs. +1.8 kg) in young healthy men doing resistance training and consuming 1.4 g/kg BW/day dietary protein evenly distributed across three meals per day compared to an uneven distribution of identical daily protein intake. This is a simple method to help preserve lean muscle mass as we age. If you find after designing your meals that one meal contains a little more protein than the others, you could schedule that meal to follow your daily exercise. There is a potential advantage to eating your higher protein meal after exercise to increase MPS according to this study [Moore, DR, et al., 2009].

The essential branched-chain amino acid, leucine, is required to trigger MPS along with an adequate dose of 'complete' protein. Complete proteins contain all nine of the essential amino acids and the twelve non-essential amino acids in the same relative proportions found in human tissues. As you may know, animal-sourced proteins are complete proteins and are very low in dietary carbohydrate whereas many whole-food plant-sourced proteins are incomplete proteins and are accompanied by more dietary carbohydrates. Low-carbohydrate, plant-sourced protein powders are an option for those who follow a vegan lifestyle. Leucine acts in conjunction with insulin to stimulate MPS by way of the signaling enzyme complex called mTOR (mammalian target of rapamycin). In children and adolescents, growth hormone, and in adolescent males, testosterone, also stimulate MPS. Animal-sourced proteins that are part of a LCD have enough leucine as long as the total daily protein intake and per meal protein intake are at the levels specified in Table 4.11. Most animal-sourced proteins are ≈ 8% leucine by weight. For example, a 3.1 ounce (87 gram) portion of ribeye steak contains ≈ 26 grams of protein and ≈ 2.5 grams of leucine which is enough to maximally stimulate MPS in young persons, whereas, a 4.8 ounce (134 gram) portion of ribeye steak contains ≈ 40 grams of protein and ≈ 3.8 grams of leucine which is enough to maximally stimulate MPS in older persons..

The time between meals also influences MPS. After consuming a meal containing an adequate protein bolus, the rate of MPS increases and peaks at about 90 mins and gradually declines until MPS reaches the pre-meal rate 5 hours later. Experimental data suggest that when cellular ATP levels decline in the muscle cell as a result of the energy demand of MPS, the signal to continue MPS is turned down. Thus, any additional protein eaten after the meal and before the end of this 5-hour period will not further increase MPS [Bohé, J, et al., 2001, Wilson, GJ, et al., 2012]. Thus, spacing meals about 5 hours apart is optimal for MPS. Coincidentally, this 5-hour time span matches the duration of action of rapid-acting mealtime bolus insulin, and nearly so, short-acting regular insulin. Thus, 5–6 hours represents an optimal time between meals for those with T1D.

Types of Dietary Fat in a Low-Carbohydrate Diet

Since the majority of our energy needs on a LCD comes from dietary fat, we should be familiar with this macronutrient. Fat takes two forms in the body: fatty acids and triglycerides. Triglycerides are simply three fatty acids bound to a glycerol molecule and are the transport and storage form of fat. Fatty acids are long carbon chains combined with hydrogen and oxygen and come in three varieties: saturated fatty acids (SFA), monounsaturated fatty acids (MUFA), and polyunsaturated fatty acids (PUFA). SFA have no double bonds between carbon atoms, MUFA have one double bond, and PUFA have more than one double bond. PUFA are further categorized as omega-6, or n-6, and omega-3, or n-3, which indicates where the first carbon-carbon double bond is located relative to the terminal (omega) end of the fatty acid, i.e., the third or sixth, in this case. When following a LCD, most of one's dietary fat intake should come from SFA and MUFA found in LCD foods like meat, fish, poultry, eggs, cheese, olives, avocado, and many others.

For years we were told to limit the amount of SFA in our diets to less than 10% of total daily calories and total dietary fat to less than 30% of total daily calories to prevent CVD. We now know this was based on a hypothesis that was never confirmed to be correct in multiple large clinical trials [Harcombe, Z, et al., 2016, Ravnskov, U, et al., 2014]. The advice to limit dietary fat and replace the calories with dietary carbohydrate and sugar is deleterious to most, especially those with insulin resistance, metabolic syndrome, and diabetes. The liver converts some of the dietary carbohydrate into SFA, primarily palmitic acid (C18) and lesser amounts of stearic acid (C16), in a process called de novo lipogenesis [Volk, BM, et al., 2014]. These SFA can be deposited in the liver causing NAFLD or are packaged into very low density lipoproteins (VLDL) for transport through the bloodstream which can result in hypertriglyceridemia because insulin resistant fat cells are unable to store more triglycerides. After many years, atherosclerosis and CVD can develop (see Chapter 11), the very disease we are supposed to be preventing with the LFHCD! A LCD can improve or resolve insulin resistance and prevent or reverse both NAFLD and hypertriglyceridemia [Mardinoglu, A, et al., 2018].

Essential and Conditionally Essential Fatty Acids

Alpha-linolenic acid (ALA), an omega-3 fatty acid (n-3), and linoleic acid (LA), an omega-6 fatty acid (n-6), are essential fatty acids, meaning they can't be synthesized by humans from other nutrients and must be obtained from dietary sources. The long-chain n-3 fatty acids, eicosapentaenoic acid (EPA) and docosahexaenoic acid (DHA), can be synthesized from ALA, but due to low conversion efficiency, are considered to be conditionally essential fatty acids, meaning they should be obtained from foods in the diet for optimal health.

The European Food Safety Authority (EFSA) recommends the following dietary intakes: ALA 0.5% and LA 4% of total daily calories, and of EPA and DHA combined, 250 mg/day. The American Heart Association recommends 500 mg/day of EPA and DHA combined, for those without CVD, and 1,000 mg/day for those with CVD. Cold-water fish including salmon, salmon roe, sardines, herring, mackerel, whitefish, and oysters, to name a few, are good sources of EPA and DHA. Because we can convert only 3% of the ALA found in flaxseed oil, walnuts, chia seeds, and other plants into EPA and DHA, we should not rely solely on these foods as a source of EPA and DHA. Vegetarians and vegans can get EPA and DHA from supplements made from microalgae, which is the dietary source of n-3 PUFA in fish. Because EPA and DHA are stored in fat, you do not necessarily need to eat seafood daily. What is important is to get at least 1,750 mg/week of EPA and DHA combined. For example, eating six ounces of salmon twice a week provides 2,290 mg of EPA and DHA combined, which exceeds the minimum requirement. LA is present in numerous foods and in sufficient quantities that it is easy to meet the RDA for this essential nutrient.

Why Avoiding Vegetable Oils May Improve Health

Wesson cooking oil (deodorized cottonseed oil) was first produced in 1899 and Crisco (partially-hydrogenated cottonseed oil) in 1911 marking more than 100 years of exposure to these non-food compounds. Increasing LA intake without also increasing EPA and DHA intake may increase the risk of CVD and death [Ramsden, CE, et al., 2010]. Excessive LA relative to EPA and DHA intake can induce direct toxic effects to the endothelial cells lining our blood vessels causing chronic inflammation and CVD [DiNicolantonio, JJ, et al., 2018]. While our immune system initiates a beneficial acute inflammatory response to defend and repair our tissues from bacteria, viruses, toxins, and injuries, chronic inflammation, from dietary factors like PUFA and sugar, causes ongoing deleterious tissue injury and repair. This can be avoided by staying away from processed and restaurant food, both of which use vegetable oils. Both the high temperature and duration of heating vegetable oils used to fry foods results in the formation of oxidized PUFA and compounds such as aldehydes which are toxic to humans [Teicholz, N, 2010]. Aldehydes react with biomolecules such as proteins and DNA, disrupting multiple cell functions including gene expression and causing tissue injury [Uchida, K, 2003].

This review article [Patterson, E, et al., 2012] discusses the health implications of consuming large amounts of n-6 PUFA from vegetable oils and inadequate amounts of n-3 PUFA from fish. "Increases in the ratio of n-6 : n-3 PUFA, characteristic of the Western diet, could potentiate inflammatory processes and consequently predispose to or exacerbate many inflammatory diseases. The change in ratio and increase in n-6 PUFA consumption change the production of important mediators and regulators of inflammation and immune responses towards a proinflammatory profile. Chronic conditions such as CVD, diabetes, obesity, rheumatoid arthritis, and inflammatory bowel disease (IBD) are all associated with increased production of prostaglandin E_2 (PGE2), leukotriene B4 (LTB4), thromboxane A2 (TXA2), interleukin-1β (IL-1β), interleukin-6 (IL-6), and tumor necrosis factor-α (TNF-α), whereby the production of these factors increases with increased dietary intake of n-6 PUFA and decreased dietary intake of n-3 PUFA. In conclusion, the unbalanced dietary consumption of n-6 : n-3 PUFA is detrimental to human health, and so the impact of dietary supplementation with n-3 PUFA upon the alleviation of inflammatory diseases, more specifically, NAFLD needs to be more thoroughly investigated."

Following a Low-Carbohydrate Diet While Traveling

Traveling, whether for business or pleasure, is quite challenging and at times difficult for those with T1D especially when following a LCD and seeking normal blood sugars. These challenges include the ubiquity of high-carbohydrate foods in restaurants, hotels, airports, airplanes, and so on. It really takes an effort to avoid all of the pitfalls of eating out when traveling simply because of the usual high-carbohydrate offerings and the unknown additions of sugar and starches to foods. Quantifying intake is also difficult when eating out unless one is willing to use a kitchen scale (awkward). Traveling also results in time-zone changes which affects our sleep pattern, circadian rhythm, and the timing of insulin doses in relation to our body's insulin needs. Eating the same meal day to day may be difficult and a compromise would be to keep all the macronutrients constant day to day by using an app like cronometer.com. I present three possible solutions to sourcing food when traveling: food you take with you, food you buy at a grocery store after you arrive, and food you eat at a restaurant.

Taking food with you may seem strange to some, but packing your food in your carry-on or checked-bag works quite well especially when traveling domestically in the U.S. Raw or pre-cooked food can be transported in plastic containers and cooked or reheated in a microwave at your destination. When traveling domestically in the U.S., check the TSA website about specific regulations that pertain to food at https://www.tsa.gov/travel/security-screening/whatcanibring/food. When traveling internationally, check the customs website for the country you will be visiting. Many countries have restrictions on what foods you can bring into their country. Don't travel with food that violates their rules, or plan to eat it on the airplane before you arrive, otherwise customs will confiscate your food. Cooked meat and jerky travel well and you can freeze it before leaving home. Meat, fish, oysters, and chicken packaged in cans or vacuumed-packed plastic bags travel well. Hard-boiled eggs, nuts & seeds, precut raw vegetables, and berries are good choices as well. Travel by car is much easier and I have packed an ice chest with all the food I need for a week of vacation.

Buying food in grocery stores is another good option when traveling especially if staying there for three or more days. We often get a room with a kitchenette that is like being at home. I can buy my usual foods and prepare them in my usual way. If my destination hotel does not have a kitchenette, I have brought an 8" non-stick cooking pan and a single hot plate to cook my meals. Many hotels have microwave ovens which work well for cooking and reheating without having to bring your own hot plate and pan. I also buy nuts, cheese, nonstarchy vegetables, raw, cooked, or frozen, and eat them as is or heat them up in the hotel microwave. I have done this for a week at a time and it works pretty well. Although eating the same meals you were eating at home is ideal, it may be difficult to find the same foods in the new grocery store. Just find the closest items you can and stick with the same meals at your new destination.

Eating in restaurants is convenient, but you have very little control over the ingredients especially if you order directly from the menu. Restaurants often add sugar and starches to savory recipes that most would not have anticipated. This can certainly result in a high blood sugar after the meal. When ordering at a restaurant, I look at the menu just to see what sorts of foods they must keep in the kitchen. Then I simply ask for a specified quantity of meat, chicken, eggs, or fish and either a nonstarchy vegetable or small salad without dressing (except juice from a lemon and olive oil). Dishes with multiple ingredients increase the likelihood of getting something you don't expect. In order to know the BID needed, you will have to order foods that closely match the macronutrients you have been eating at home. You can estimate the macronutrients with cronometer.com on a cell phone or just 'wing it.'

The Low-Carbohydrate Diet for Vegans and Vegetarians

A recent Gallup poll in the U.S. found that 5% of respondents identified themselves as following a vegetarian and 3% a vegan diet. Achieving normal blood sugars and improved body composition with lower insulin doses while preserving lean muscle mass requires adequate protein intake and low carbohydrate intake. This is fairly straightforward when following a vegetarian eating pattern due the ability to include eggs and dairy foods, but doing so following a vegan eating pattern is more challenging. This is due to the fact that vegan protein sources are typically higher in carbohydrate content than animal-based protein sources. Use of low-carbohydrate, plant-based, protein powder is one solution. A vegan LCD/VLCD should be carefully planned to meet not only macro- and micronutrient requirements, but also the proper balance of amino acids. Soy and quinoa, and pea (low in methionine) combined with rice protein (low in lysine), protein powders are complete proteins and come in low-carbohydrate versions. See these articles for more guidance on this topic at https://blog.virtahealth.com/vegan-vegetarian-low-carb-keto/ and https://www.dietdoctor.com/low-carb/vegan. Carrie Diulus, MD (@cadiulus on twitter) has T1D and maintains normal blood sugars on a vegan diet using a DIY artificial pancreas.

The Low-Carbohydrate Diet for Carnivores

The carnivore diet is an elimination diet that is useful in determining if one or more physical signs, symptoms, or diseases is caused by an intolerance to one or more foods. Anecdotal reports of improvements in numerous physical and mental symptoms and improvement or reversal of various diseases have been reported on the internet by following a carnivore diet composed exclusively of animal foods. Autoimmune diseases are frequently reported as improving on the carnivore elimination diet including rheumatoid arthritis and inflammatory bowel diseases like ulcerative colitis and Crohn's disease. Since humans can also be intolerant of some animal foods, most notably eggs and dairy products, if a carnivore diet is being used as an elimination diet, eggs and dairy products, should initially be excluded as well. If the physical signs, symptoms, or diseases improve or resolve, then previously excluded foods can be added back into the diet, one at a time. The reintroduction of foods into the diet should be separated by several weeks to allow time for physical signs or symptoms to return if the latest food added back is a culprit food. The primary reason for adding back additional foods is to provide essential and conditionally essential nutrients. For many, reintroducing foods will also make the diet more sustainable long-term which is very important for those with T1D. Some of the essential nutrients found in inadequate amounts in beef (skeletal muscle) include omega-3 fatty acids, EPA and DHA, vitamin B5 (pantothenic acid), biotin, choline, vitamin B9 (folate), vitamin A, vitamin C, vitamin D (but can be made from adequate sun exposure), vitamin K1, calcium, molybdenum, and manganese. To help fill-in any nutritional gaps, other animal foods that can be added back, one at a time, include pork, organ meats (offal), eggs, dairy, oily fish (salmon, herring, mackerel), sardines, and oysters. Plant foods can also be added back, one at a time, to supply many of these essential nutrients as well. That said, some following a carnivore diet have found by trial and error that they are intolerant of all plant foods and do not plan on adding back any additional plant foods to avoid suffering the problems that their removal had previously resolved. In these cases, a special effort should be expended to find animal sources of all the essential nutrients or use vitamin/mineral supplements. I think making the effort to get as many of the essential nutrients as possible is an insurance policy against long-term nutritional deficiencies as mentioned previously in reference to Dr. Bruce Ames's triage hypothesis [Ames, BN, 2006].

Adding More Flexibility to Meals

Once blood sugars have normalized, you can experiment with varying meals more often than once weekly with constant macronutrients. If this maintains normal blood sugars, you can experiment with estimating meals by eye rather than adding up macronutrients. Making your diet more flexible will make it easier to sustain. Doing so after achieving normal blood sugars will give you direct feedback as to exactly how much variability you can incorporate into your meal plan. If your blood sugar control deteriorates, you will know the last change you made was likely the reason.

Sample Day of Eating a Very Low-Carbohydrate Diet

Using cronometer.com, I took my goal macronutrient totals to design three meals/day.

Goal carbohydrate grams = 39 grams/day ÷ 3 meals/day = 13 grams/meal.

Goal protein grams = 167 grams/day ÷ 3 meals/day = 56 grams/meal.

Goal fat grams = 211 grams/day ÷ 3 meals/day = 70 grams/meal.

The menu is shown at the top and the macronutrients (grams) and micronutrients (% RDA) are shown in the bottom of Table 4.12.

Table 4.12 — Sample Day of Eating a Very Low-Carbohydrate Diet

Breakfast	Amt	Lunch	Amt	Dinner	Amt
Large Eggs	4	Salmon	168 g	Beef, 80% lean	168 g
Bacon	40 g	Sauerkraut	75 g		
Cheddar cheese	28 g	Cheddar cheese	28 g	Cheddar cheese	28 g
Pistachios	12 g	Pistachios	12 g	Pistachios	12 g
Keto Mousse	52 g	Keto Mousse	52 g	Keto Mousse	52 g
		Butter, salted	21 g	Butter, salted	7 g
Kale, raw	50 g	Kale, raw	50 g	Kale, raw	50 g
Total Carbs	40 g	Riboflavin	269%	Vitamin E	130%

Fiber	18 g	Niacin	208%	Vitamin K	527%
Total Fat	218 g	Pantothenic Acid	190%	Calcium	134%
Fat, Monos	75 g	Pyridoxine	230%	Copper	249%
Fat, Polys	28 g	Cobalamin	552%	Iron	206%
Fat, n-3	6 g	Biotin	141%	Magnesium	88%
Fat, n-6	21 g	Choline	175%	Manganese	167%
Fat, Saturated	93 g	Folate	89%	Phosphorus	313%
Total Protein	169 g	Lutein+Zeaxanthin	94%	Potassium	103%
Leucine	8.1 g	Vitamin A	385%	Selenium	435%
Ketogenic Ratio	1.71	Vitamin C	173%	Sodium	177%
Thiamine	148%	Vitamin D	136%	Zinc	202%
% Calories, Carbs	6%	% Calories, Fat	70%	% Calories, Protein	24%

Note: I take these supplements: MgCl, 150 mg/day, Vitamin C 180 mg/day, Vitamin B12 0.5 mg twice weekly, Vitamin D 5,000 IU 4x/week, Creatine 2 grams/day. Other meals I rotate through have more folate, such that I meet or exceed 100% of RDA.

I abstained from eating dessert from 2011 until August 2019 due to my dislike of the taste of artificial sweeteners. By chance, I came across this YouTube video from Megha and Matt at Keto Connect, https://www.youtube.com/watch?v=Gqo8NTp28pc, and decided to try it. I replaced the mascarpone cheese with cream cheese and added MCT and coconut oils to increase the calories and my ketone levels. I now have a chocolate dessert I can enjoy without adversely affecting my blood sugars. If you need to lose body fat, you can remove the MCT and coconut oil or find a less calorically-dense dessert recipe.

Keto Chocolate Mousse Recipe

1. In a storage bowl, melt coconut oil (50 grams) in microwave for 15 secs.
2. Add MCT Oil (50 grams),
3. Add 10 tbsp of Shiloh Farms™ non-alkalinized cocoa powder (50 grams),
4. Add 1 cup heavy whipping cream (235 grams),
5. Add Vanilla Sweet Drops™ (liquid stevia) (19 grams) and mix with spoon or electric mixer,
6. Add 16 oz of Philadelphia™ cream cheese at room temperature or heat on high in microwave for 15 secs per 8 oz bar to soften (454 grams), mix ingredients with spoon first, then use electric mixer,
7. Add 84 grams raw sunflower seeds,
8. Add 84 grams raw pecans,
9. Add 84 grams raw hazelnuts, then stir with spoon,
10. Store in refrigerator for up to 7 days. It can be frozen and thawed later.

Note: The 19 grams of liquid stevia (< 1 gram/serving) in this recipe does not make it taste sweet, rather it masks the bitterness of the cocoa powder. If you have difficulty with quitting sugar, I suggest not further increasing the amount of liquid stevia because artificial sweeteners can fuel a sugar addiction. The total weight of the recipe is 1,110 grams, and when divided by 21 meals, yields 53 grams/meal.
Total Carbs = 103 g or 5 g/meal (6.5% of calories).

Total Fiber = 42 g or 2 g/meal.
Total Fat = 501 g or 24 g/meal (86.9% of calories).
Total Protein = 82 g or 4 g/meal (6.6% of calories).
Total Calories = 5,090 kcal or 242 kcal/meal.
Ketogenic Ratio = 2.43.

5 – Insulin Preparations, Dosing & Delivery

"The diabetic who knows the most, lives the longest."
Elliott P. Joslin, MD, America's first diabetologist.

Good, better, best. Never let it rest. 'Til your good is better, and your better, is best."
St. Jerome, Latin priest.

"The greater danger for most of us lies not in setting our aim too high and falling short;
but in setting our aim too low, and achieving our mark."
Michelangelo, Italian sculptor, painter, architect and poet of the High Renaissance.

This chapter provides important information about selecting insulin preparations, the proper use of insulin, modes of delivery, and dosing of insulin. Elliott P. Joslin, MD cautioned both patients and doctors that, "Insulin is a remedy that is primarily for the wise and not the foolish." What he meant was that insulin has a narrow therapeutic window such that the range of insulin doses that result in a normal blood sugar is quite narrow. When too much or too little insulin is given, both can have serious consequences. In short, the dose of insulin has to be 'just right.' This is what makes managing T1D so challenging and why I am grateful that I have managed to find a solution that I can share with you.

Intensive Insulin Therapy

The Diabetes Control and Complications Trial (DCCT) [The DCCT Research Group, 1993b] enrolled 1,441 patients with T1D at 29 centers from 1983 to 1989 who were followed for a mean of 6.5 years to test the hypothesis that intensive insulin therapy with intent to normalize glycemic control would lessen or prevent diabetic complications of the eyes (retinopathy), kidneys (nephropathy), and nerves (neuropathy) compared to conventional insulin therapy. Prior to initiation of this randomized controlled trial (RCT), diabetes experts debated whether poor glycemic control was the primary cause of long-term diabetic complications as apposed to other factors, e.g., duration of diabetes, age, genetic factors, etc. The investigators were also concerned about the development of hypoglycemia and weight gain by simply intensifying insulin therapy. Two groups of adolescents and young adults were randomized, those with recently diagnosed T1D without retinopathy, the primary-prevention cohort (n = 726), and those with pre-existing retinopathy, the secondary-intervention cohort (n = 715). The TDID was higher with intensive insulin therapy, 0.71 IU/kg/day, compared to conventional insulin therapy, 0.65 IU/kg/day [Braffett, BH, et al., 2019a]. Intensive insulin therapy (three or more insulin doses per day, adjusted per diet, exercise, and blood sugar results) reduced the mean blood glucose from 231 mg/dl (12.8 mM) to 155 mg/dl (8.6 mM) and reduced the development of retinopathy by 76%, of neuropathy by 69%, and of microalbuminuria by 34% in the primary-prevention cohort subjects compared to conventional insulin therapy (one or two insulin doses per day, usually fixed doses). In the secondary-intervention cohort, intensive therapy slowed the progression of retinopathy by 54% and reduced the development of neuropathy by 57% and of microalbuminuria by 43%. As was feared, intensive insulin therapy was associated with a 3-fold higher incidence of severe hypoglycemia (62 vs. 19 episodes requiring assistance per 100-patient years) and a mean gain of 4.6 kg bodyweight after 5 years. The intensive insulin therapy group was counseled by dietitians to follow the LFHCD with 45–55% of daily calories from carbohydrates and up to 25% of daily carbohydrates from simple sugars [The DCCT Research Group, 1993a]. In my opinion, this dietary advice likely explains why the intensive insulin therapy group was unable to achieve normal blood sugars, the stated goal of the study, and suffered from severe hypoglycemia and weight gain. However, the DCCT did demonstrate that improving glycemic control did significantly reduce long-term diabetic complications. An RCT should be conducted using a LCD with intensive insulin therapy and consistent meals, exercise, and adequate sleep day to day as described in this book to assess the beneficial, as well as potential adverse, outcomes.

Most of those with T1D use intensive insulin therapy consisting of basal intermediate or long-acting insulin designed for between-meal and overnight insulin needs and rapid- or short-acting bolus insulin for meals and blood sugar corrections with and/or between meals. Rapid-acting insulin analogs were originally developed to accommodate the rapid rise in post-meal blood glucose from the dietary carbohydrate content of the LFHCD as well as the rapid stomach-emptying and nutrient absorption that results from the loss of amylin secretion from the lack of β-cells in those with T1D. Some who follow a LCD find that a rapid-acting insulin analog matches the timing of nutrient absorption despite the lower dietary carbohydrate intake, while others have relatively delayed nutrient absorption that can result in hypoglycemia when using a rapid-acting insulin analog and find that short-acting regular insulin better matches the timing of nutrient absorption.

Exogenous Insulin Preparations for Type 1 Diabetes

Exogenous insulin can be administered by four different routes: inhaled, injected, pumped, and added to dialysis fluid (for peritoneal dialysis patients only). Inhaled insulin provides the most rapid absorption and insulin action. The only inhaled insulin currently on the market in the U.S. is Afrezza. It is relatively new, I have not used it, nor prescribed it to patients. There are two potential problems with inhaled insulin: 1) it can only be administered in 4 IU dosage increments, and 2) its absorption into the bloodstream from the lungs is quite variable causing variable blood glucose responses. The authors of this review article [Pettus, J, et al., 2018] state that 4 IU of Afrezza behaves "roughly similar to 2.5 IU of a rapid-acting insulin analog." This dosage increment would likely be too large to be usable by most of those following a LCD. I will defer further discussion of insulin administered via inhalation or dialysate fluid to the prescribing physician.

Injected insulin comes in four forms based on duration of action: 1) rapid-acting insulin analogs, 2) short-acting regular insulin, 3) intermediate-acting NPH insulin, and 4) long-acting basal insulin analogs. You and your healthcare provider will decide which insulin preparations are best for you, but I will provide you with some information about them to help you understand the rationale for choosing one preparation over another. Four important characteristics of each insulin preparation are listed in Table 5.1, 1) its time to onset of action, 2) its time to peak action, 3) its duration of action, and 4) its day-to-day variability of action.

Table 5.1 — Insulin Preparation Action Times & Variability

Insulin Preparation U100	Onset	Peak	Duration	Instructions and Notes	Day-to-day Variability
Afrezza, Inhaled insulin	12–15 mins	1 hour	2.5–3 hours	Minimum 4 IU dose, and in 4 IU increments.	Moderate
Glulisine (Apidra), Lispro (Humalog), Aspart (Novolog)	5–15 mins	1–2 hours	4–5 hours	If pre-meal blood sugar low or when not in control of time meal arrives, take after meal, otherwise take at start of meal.	Low
Regular Human Insulin (Humulin R, Novolin R)	20–60 mins	2–4 hours	8–10 hours	Inject 30 mins before meal. Inject at start of meal when not in control of time meal arrives.	Moderate
NPH insulin (Humulin N, Novolin N)	1–2 hours	4–8 hours	10–12 hours	Taken 2–4 times daily, at same times of day, each day. Caution: nocturnal hypoglycemia.	High
Detemir (Levemir)	1–2 hours	Minimal	12–20 hours	Take once or twice daily, same time of day, 12 hours apart.	Moderate
Glargine (Lantus)	1–2 hours	Minimal	20–24 hours	Take once or twice daily at same time of day.	Moderate
Degludec (Tresiba)	1–2 hours	None	> 42 hours	Take once daily at same time of day.	Low

Note 1: The table above is an abbreviated list of insulin preparations currently on the market. I have specifically excluded all of the

concentrated insulin preparations, U200, U300, U500, which are not appropriate for those with T1D following a LCD. I have also omitted numerous pre-mixed insulin preparations composed of NPH and short- or rapid-acting insulins because their pharmacokinetic properties rarely match the insulin needs of those with T1D following a LCD.

Note 2: The assessments of day-to-day variability are impressions I gleaned from my review of the medical literature. Technically, this attribute is called the 'within-subject variability' measured using pharmacodynamic and pharmacokinetic data from multiple different studies.

Use of Rapid-Acting and Short-Acting Bolus Insulin

Most persons with T1D use one of three rapid-acting bolus insulin analog preparations (glulisine (Apidra), lispro (Humalog), aspart (Novolog)) for meals and blood sugar corrections as shown in Table 5.1. The more rapid onset of action is produced by substituting or rearranging amino acids in the insulin molecule, hence the name insulin analog. The amino acid alterations primarily affect the rate of absorption into the bloodstream leaving its effect on the insulin receptor unchanged. These insulin preparations have similar half-lives as shown in Table 5.2 and therefore will produce similar post-meal blood sugar responses. The half-life is the time required for half of the injected insulin to be absorbed from the site of injection and cleared from the bloodstream which determines the time of onset of action, time to peak action, and duration of action. Some may find that one rapid-acting insulin preparation better matches the timing of their nutrient absorption and thus results in normal blood sugars when properly dosed. Trying different insulin preparations is the best way to determine which is best for you. Short-acting regular insulin is identical to human insulin, but when injected into the subcutaneous fat, has a slower onset of action, later peak of action, and longer duration of action than either rapid-acting insulin analogs or endogenous insulin secreted by the β-cells. Short-acting regular insulin also has more day-to-day variability in action compared to rapid-acting insulin analogs [Ganiats, T, 2006]. Despite this potential for day-to-day variability in action, short-acting regular insulin may, in fact, be a useful insulin preparation for some following a LCD if it more accurately matches one's rate of nutrient absorption due to the lower carbohydrate or higher protein content of a LCD or due to diabetic gastroparesis.

Use of Intermediate-Acting NPH Insulin

NPH (Neutral Protamine Hagedorn) insulin, introduced in 1950, is the only intermediate-acting basal insulin. NPH is human insulin with protamine and zinc added to delay its absorption into the bloodstream. When NPH is used twice daily as a basal insulin, it does result in more nocturnal hypoglycemia than the long-acting basal insulin analogs. This effect can be mitigated if taken every 6 hours, before three evenly-spaced meals and at bedtime, in which case, bolus insulin is usually not needed when following a LCD. I have not tested this strategy myself with a LCD to achieve normal blood sugars, but it is worth a try if the cost of insulin analogs is prohibitive for you.

Use of Long-Acting Basal Insulin Analogs

Basal insulin serves to provide a steady source of insulin between meals and while sleeping. Basal insulin begins working 1–2 hours after injection and reaches a steady-state level after ≈ 2 hours for detemir (Levemir), ≈ 6 hours for glargine (Lantus), and ≈ 8 hours for degludec (Tresiba) after the initial injection. The longer the duration of action, the less variation in insulin release will occur during each 24-hour period. Over the years, the pharmaceutical industry has been working on developing longer-acting basal insulins for this reason. The basal insulin analog with the longest duration of action and least day-to-day variability in action is degludec (Tresiba) as shown in Table 5.1. Basal insulin analogs should be taken once or twice daily with one dose at bedtime and for detemir (Levemir) and NPH (Humulin N), the second dose 12 hours later. Glargine (Lantus), or any basal insulin for that matter, can be taken twice daily if doing so further improves your glycemic control. Taking basal insulin twice daily, with half the daily dose in each injection, will reduce the apparent variation in insulin appearance in the bloodstream during a 24-hour period. Of course, if taking basal insulin once daily works well, there is no reason to take it more often. I experimented with taking glargine (Lantus) 2- and 3-times daily with multiple different dosing schemes and did not see any improvement by doing so. The basal insulin dose taken at bedtime is adjusted to hit your target fasting blood sugar while still avoiding hypoglycemia during the night. From my experience actually using all of these basal insulins, I would rank the currently available U100 basal insulin preparations in terms of providing the best blood sugar results as follows: 1) degludec (Tresiba), 2) glargine (Lantus), 3) detemir (Levemir), and 4) NPH insulin. That said, the difference between degludec (Tresiba) and glargine (Lantus) was small, in my experience, and the extra cost of degludec (Tresiba) may not be justified for some. My observations generally agree with information found in the medical literature [Haahr, H, et al., 2014, Heise, T, et al., 2018].

Variability in Insulin Action

This review article [Ganiats, T, 2006] states: "A major limitation of both regular human insulin and NPH is that they do not accurately reproduce physiologic insulin secretion. For example, regular human insulin has a slow onset of action and a delayed peak of action. NPH exhibits a significant peak in action and a relatively short duration of action, both of which limit its ability to meet basal insulin needs. Moreover, both regular human insulin and NPH exhibit considerable variation within an individual patient. This variability in insulin action means that identical doses of subcutaneous insulin injections do not always lead to the same glycemic effects, even if dietary intake and physical activity are controlled. Therefore, the pharmacokinetic profiles of conventional human insulin formulations and the unpredictable nature of these profiles can result in insulin levels that are not appropriately matched to the patient's needs." The article also points out several important and correctable causes of blood glucose variability due to variability in insulin action. List 1 enumerates the consequences of variability of insulin action and why we want to minimize this variability, and List 2 enumerates the causes of variability in insulin action which can be improved with proper selection of your insulin preparation, its administration, and the consistency of your meals, exercise, and sleep. Trying different insulin preparations is a good way to determine which one will minimize your blood sugar variability from day to day.

List 1: Potential Consequences of Variability in Insulin Action.
1. Increased risk of hypoglycemia.
2. Increased weight gain associated with defensive eating to prevent hypoglycemia.
3. Changes in appetite due to fluctuations in glucose/insulin levels.
4. Reduced patient confidence in their treatment due to variability in glucose levels.
5. Increased risk of development and/or progression of diabetes complications.

6. Increased risk of mortality.

List 2: Causes of Intraindividual Variability in Insulin Action.
1. Factors related to the insulin preparation:
   - Physicochemical properties of the insulin preparation — different insulin preparations inherently result in different blood sugar variabilities which can help determine which insulin preparation is best for you. See day-to-day variability in Table 5.1.
   - Insulin comes in a range of concentrations including U100, U200, U300, and U500. U100 or diluted insulin, e.g., U20, are appropriate for those following a LCD, while U200, U300, and U500 were designed for those with insulin-resistant T2D taking large doses of insulin.
2. Factors depending on the injection conditions:
   - Depth of injection — choose the correct needle length based on the amount of subcutaneous fat you have in the location being injected. Using a needle that is too long can result in an intramuscular injection which shortens the time of onset and peak of insulin action and decreases the duration of action.
   - Anatomical site of injection — insulin is absorbed at different rates from different sites of injection: thigh, abdomen, buttocks, and arm. Frequently changing injection areas can increase variability in the blood glucose response to insulin. Conversely, rarely changing injection areas can lead to lipohypertrophy (excess subcutaneous fat accumulation) and increased blood glucose variability.
   - Delay before withdrawing the needle — you should count to 10 sec before withdrawing the needle and withdraw it very slowly to prevent insulin from leaking out of the injection site. Tell children that pain from a needle only occurs during insertion. The quicker

the insertion of the needle, the less discomfort. Once the needle has penetrated the skin, there should be no more discomfort. Some may feel a cold sensation from injecting refrigerated insulin, but it is not painful. Removing the needle slowly is not painful either.
- Blood flow in the subcutaneous tissue at the site of injection — exercising soon after insulin injections quickens the rate of insulin absorption and action and could cause hypoglycemia.

3. Factors related to the individual:
- Hypoglycemic effect — hypoglycemia can trigger counterregulatory hormone secretion that increases insulin resistance and subsequent blood sugars.
- Physical activity — exercise increases insulin sensitivity which requires less insulin post-exercise. Varying exercise from day to day will also vary insulin sensitivity from day to day resulting in increased blood sugar variability.
- Diet — varying a LCD meal from day to day results in increased blood sugar variability.

Diabetic Gastroparesis

I have not emphasized specific treatment of long-term diabetic complications in this book because I feel the fundamental and most effective treatment for diabetic complications is normalization of blood sugars. Nonetheless, one long-term complication, diabetic gastroparesis, can affect which mealtime insulin preparation works best. Diabetic gastroparesis is an autonomic neuropathy of the vagus nerve that innervates the stomach and controls its motility. Food moves through the stomach and digestive tract more slowly than normal in those with diabetic gastroparesis. This results in delayed absorption of nutrients which in turn affects the blood sugar response to the mealtime bolus insulin. Diabetic gastroparesis affects 20–50% of those with long-standing T1D [Krishnasamy, S, et al., 2018]. The symptoms of diabetic gastroparesis include nausea, vomiting, bloating, early satiety, and abdominal discomfort.

Because diabetic gastroparesis slows the rate of absorption of nutrients and the rate of rise in post-meal blood sugar, those with this condition may benefit from using short-acting regular insulin instead of a rapid-acting insulin analog. They may find when using a rapid-acting insulin analog that they develop hypoglycemia within two hours of taking it, and if they reduce the dose enough to avoid hypoglycemia, the 5-hour post-meal blood sugar reading is consistently high. Put another way, they are unable to find any dose of a rapid-acting insulin analog that results in both a normal 5-hour post-meal blood sugar and does not cause hypoglycemia. This problem can be solved by using short-acting regular insulin (Humulin R) which has a slower onset of action and longer duration of action which more closely matches the slower nutrient absorption rate in those with diabetic gastroparesis. Diabetic gastroparesis is a reversible condition as are most all of the peripheral and autonomic neurologic diabetic complications. The time required to reverse the condition varies considerably from many months to years.

Insulin-Stacking

Insulin-stacking is a term used to describe giving a dose of bolus insulin before the previous dose has completed its duration of action. In Table 5.2, the percent of bolus insulin absorbed versus time after injection is calculated using the half-life of each bolus insulin. For all the rapid-acting insulin analogs, more than 90% of the injected dose will be absorbed by five hours after injection. At the 5-hour mark, 77–90% of regular insulin will be absorbed after injection depending on which half-life is used in the calculation (see Note in Table 5.2). If meals are spaced every 5–6 hours, there will be no insulin-stacking when using rapid-acting insulin and the impact of insulin-stacking when using short-acting regular insulin will be minimal as long as the time-of-day of the meal does not vary from day to day. But, if meals are eaten at different times from day to day regardless of the bolus insulin preparation used, then insulin-stacking could occur on some days, but not others, making the blood glucose response variable. Assuming three meals are eaten per day, this means correction doses, if needed, can be added to, or subtracted from, the mealtime bolus doses. A correction dose can be taken at bedtime, if needed. If one or two meals are eaten per day, then a correction dose(s) could be given, if needed, as long as it has been five hours since the last dose and will be five hours before the next dose. If four meals are eaten per day, all of the correction doses, if needed, can be added to, or subtracted from, the four mealtime bolus doses. Thus, to avoid the variability in blood glucose due to insulin-stacking, bolus insulin should not be taken more frequently than ≈ 5 hours. One of the 'advantages' of using an insulin pump or artificial pancreas device is supposed to be the ability to give correction doses between meals to correct hyperglycemia. The pump keeps track of the 'insulin-on-board' to prevent you from giving too much by using a patented algorithm. This can cause hypoglycemia due to insulin-stacking and be avoided by giving bolus insulin no more frequently than every 5 hours.

Table 5.2 — Percent of Bolus Insulin Absorbed Versus Time After Injection

Insulin	Glulisine Apidra	Lispro Humalog	Aspart Novolog	Regular Humulin R	Regular Humulin R

Time After Injection	R1. Half-life 42 mins	R2. Half-life 54 mins	R3. Half-life 81 mins	R4. Half-life 90 mins	R3. Half-life 141 mins
1 hour	63%	54%	40%	37%	26%
2 hours	86%	79%	64%	60%	45%
3 hours	95%	90%	79%	75%	59%
4 hours	98%	95%	87%	84%	69%
5 hours	99%	98%	92%	90%	77%
6 hours	100%	99%	95%	94%	83%
7 hours	100%	100%	97%	96%	87%
8 hours	100%	100%	98%	97%	91%
9 hours	100%	100%	99%	98%	93%
10 hours	100%	100%	99%	99%	95%

R1. glulisine https://www.accessdata.fda.gov/drugsatfda_docs/label/2008/021629s015lbl.pdf

R2. lispro https://www.accessdata.fda.gov/drugsatfda_docs/label/2013/020563s115lbl.pdf

R3. aspart https://www.accessdata.fda.gov/drugsatfda_docs/label/2005/020986s033lbl.pdf

R4. regular (Humulin R) https://pi.lilly.com/us/humulin-r-pi.pdf

Note: There appears to be some discrepancy regarding the half-life of short-acting regular insulin. The Humulin R reference, R4, at the bottom of Table 5.2 indicates a half-life of 90 mins, while the aspart reference, R3, indicates a half-life of 141 mins. This may be because the manufacturer of aspart wants to indicate that aspart is a rapid-acting insulin relative to regular insulin which it could not convincingly do if it quoted a half-life of 90 mins for regular insulin and 81 mins for aspart.

Insulin Pens

Insulin pens have largely replaced syringes due to their simplicity and slightly smaller diameter needles that are more comfortable. Insulin pens have two choices for needle gauge: 31 gauge or 32 gauge, and many different lengths: from 4–13 mm. One downside to using U100 insulin pens is that you are limited to 1 IU increments. Thus if you want to be able to administer insulin in fractions of an IU, you will need to use a syringe to administer diluted insulin as described above. Insulin in pens cannot be diluted.

Insulin Syringes

There are three different sizes of insulin syringes: 3/10 ml which delivers up to 30 IU of U100 insulin, 1/2 ml which delivers up to 50 IU of U100 insulin, and 1 ml which delivers up to 100 IU of U100 insulin. You should choose the smallest syringe that is still large enough to deliver your largest dose of the day. You can also use more than one size syringe for different doses, if needed. For example, if you need 10 IU for a bolus insulin injection, use the 3/10 ml syringe. But if you need 35 IU for a bolus insulin injection, use the 1/2 ml syringe. Insulin syringes come in a range of needle lengths, 4–12.7 mm, and are usually 31-gauge. The shorter needles, 4–6 mm, are best for those who are lean (without much subcutaneous fat). The larger the gauge, the smaller the needle diameter. A 31-gauge needle has a 0.261 mm outside diameter and is thicker in diameter than a 32-gauge needle with a 0.235 mm outside diameter. The larger gauge needles are therefore more comfortable. In fact, sometimes you can't even feel the 32-gauge needle passing through the skin at all!

Injecting Insulin

When injecting insulin it is important to focus your thoughts on the task at hand and not be distracted by thinking about other things or talking to others. Carefully 1) select the correct insulin type (basal vs. bolus), 2) select the correct dose on the pen, in the syringe, or on the pump, and 3) inject it with proper technique. When injecting insulin, choose a body part that you like best. The options are upper buttocks, thigh, abdomen, and the back of the upper arm. Insulin is absorbed from different sites of injection at slightly different rates. Injecting in the same body area for at least several weeks at a time will reduce variability in insulin absorption. Using two fingers to gently 'pinch' a small mound of skin helps to avoid injecting into the underlying muscle. This is most easily done on the thighs and abdomen. Inadvertently injecting insulin into muscle will increase the rate of absorption and could cause hypoglycemia. Keeping the needle in place after injection for a count of 10 and slowly withdrawing it helps to reduce leakage of insulin from the skin so that you get the intended dose. Tell children that pain from a needle only occurs during insertion. The quicker the insertion, the less discomfort. Once the needle has penetrated the skin, there should be no more discomfort. The coolness of refrigerated insulin can be felt, but it is not painful. Removing the needle slowly is not painful either. Sometimes the injection site will bleed because the needle penetrated a small vein. This is not a problem. Apply mild pressure to the site for a count of 10. You may notice a bruise at this location in the next few days, but this also is not a problem. Those who take blood-thinning medications will have larger bruises. Avoid injecting into a small area repeatedly as this can lead to lipohypertrophy, an increase in subcutaneous fat accumulation. This occurs because the high concentration of insulin at the injection site stimulates fat cells to take-up and retain fat. Lipohypertrophy should be avoided because it causes increased day-to-day variability in insulin absorption, and thus, the blood sugar response. Lipohypertrophy can be avoided by moving the injection sites around in the same body region. It is also important to devise a system to avoid forgetting to take insulin injections. As conscientious as I am, I have forgotten to take my insulin on numerous occasions over the years. But in the past few years, I have not missed any doses of metformin or insulin by placing the next dose of metformin and an unfilled insulin syringe with a sign on the kitchen counter. I also use alarms on my electronic devices as a reminder that it is time for the next meal, metformin dose, insulin dose, and exercise session.

Care of Insulin Vials and Pens

Insulin should be refrigerated whenever possible because it will take longer to use a given quantity of insulin due to the lower insulin doses when following a LCD. When traveling or otherwise taking your insulin outside your home, I suggest using the FRIO® insulin cooling cases for insulin vials and pens. They contain beads that once soaked in water will allow the water to evaporate keeping the insulin cool without the need for a power source. Even though the insulin manufacturers say it is 'okay' to store insulin at room temperature for a month while using it, keeping it cool will help it last longer than a month.

Dosing Basal Insulin

Determining the correct basal insulin dose begins with the TDID which is usually based on bodyweight. Initial TDID are typically in the range of

0.4–1.0 IU/kg per day in adults on a typical LFHCD although higher and lower doses are certainly possible. On a LFHCD, for children 9 months to 2 years of age, a reasonable TDID is 0.25–0.5 IU/kg/day, children age 1–6 years ≈ 0.5–0.6 IU/kg/day, children age > 7 years until the onset of puberty, ≈ 0.75 IU/kg/day, and during puberty ≈ 0.75–1.5 IU/kg/day of insulin is typical [Beck, JK, et al., 2015]. On a LFHCD, basal insulin requirements are usually ≈ 50% of the TDID. On a LCD, it is important to understand that the TDID in children, adolescents, and adults are significantly lower, about half the dose required on a LFHCD, and the basal insulin requirements are usually 60–80%, instead of ≈ 50% of the TDID due to the lower BID requirements. In this survey [Lennerz, BS, et al., 2018] of 316 persons with T1D following a VLCD, the mean TDID was ≈ 0.40 IU/kg/day of which ≈ 64% was basal insulin. Using these figures as an example, a person with T1D on a LCD weighing 70 kg would need ≈ 0.40 IU/kg/day × 70 kg = 28 IU/day. Of that, 28 IU/day × 0.64 = 18 IU/day is basal insulin. Those with recently diagnosed T1D or LADA still in the 'honeymoon' phase may need significantly less insulin and may be able to normalize blood sugars with a LCD and basal insulin alone. Once you find a basal insulin dose that maintains blood sugar in the normal range through the night, try to keep it stable from day to day, which will make predicting BID easier. If a change in basal insulin dose is needed due to abnormal nocturnal or fasting blood sugars, increase the dose by 5–10% for high blood sugars or decrease the dose by 10–15% for low blood sugars with 3–5 days between dose changes until a normal nocturnal and fasting blood sugar pattern is again achieved. For example, if your basal insulin dose is 20 IU/day and you need to reduce it by 10–15% for low nocturnal or fasting blood sugars, multiply 20 IU by 0.85–0.9 to get 17–18 IU. Likewise, if you need to increase it by 5–10% for high nocturnal or fasting blood sugars, multiply 20 IU by 1.05–1.1 to get 21–22 IU. Always remember that hypoglycemia is more dangerous than short-term high blood sugars which is the rationale for the larger percentage reduction in basal insulin dose for low blood sugars compared to the smaller percentage increase for high blood sugars.

I have made the mistake of adjusting my basal insulin dose nightly to compensate for a high or low bedtime blood sugar. This is not helpful because any change in the basal dose will affect every subsequent blood sugar reading for the next 3–5 days. In order to compensate for different bedtime blood sugars without having to alter the bedtime basal insulin dose, I have found that giving a small bedtime correction BID, if needed, is effective when seeking normal blood sugars. If the bedtime blood sugar is below your target range, correct it with dextrose. Always start with a tiny BID and adjust it depending on the blood sugar results. Initially checking blood sugar four hours after a bedtime BID is also a good idea. Assuming a near-normal bedtime blood sugar, if the bedtime correction BID exceeds 10–15% of the bedtime basal insulin dose, the odds of developing nocturnal hypoglycemia increase, and an increase in the basal insulin dose and reduction in the bedtime correction BID will reduce the likelihood of hypoglycemia.

Dosing Bolus Insulin

Determining the correct mealtime or correction BID is the most challenging aspect of managing T1D, especially on a LFHCD, but also on a LCD. Even the most advanced technology, the artificial pancreas, is unable to determine the mealtime BID and relies on the user to input the dose and the pump subsequently adjusts the basal rate to compensate for any mismatch between the meal and BID. My strategy for many years was to make a 'guess' after looking at the pre- and post-meal blood sugar readings and insulin doses on previous days while keeping my food choices and meal portions about the same from day to day. Although this approach was likely better than some other conceivable solutions, I was never satisfied with my results. Most of the hypoglycemic episodes I experienced occurred after meals. They typically occurred 2.5–3 hours after the mealtime insulin dose. Thus, I routinely checked my blood sugar 3 hours after each dose to see if my blood sugar was low. It was only after I experienced a marked reduction in hypoglycemia by using the strategies detailed in this book, did I change my post-meal blood sugar checks to 5.5 hours after breakfast and lunch and 4.5 hours after dinner.

As soon as you begin reducing meal carbohydrate content, the BID will need to be reduced. Start with a low BID for each meal, e.g., 25–50% of previous doses. Then on each subsequent day, adjust the dose based on both the previous day's change in blood sugar and the current day's pre-meal blood sugar. At the end of this chapter, I will show you a mathematical method to estimate each BID. Mealtime bolus insulin should generally be taken with each meal, although when on a LCD, there may certainly be times when a BID should be withheld. Rapid-acting insulin is usually taken at the start of eating a meal, but could be taken before preparing your own meal if the blood sugar is at or above your target and you know the meal will be ready in less than 20 mins. If the pre-meal blood sugar is below your target blood glucose without any symptoms, I suggest postponing taking rapid-acting insulin until after you have eaten the meal to prevent hypoglycemia. If you are having symptomatic hypoglycemia, it should be treated immediately with dextrose as usual. The same guidelines apply to short-acting regular insulin, except delayed by 15 mins due to its delayed onset of action. When you are not in control of preparing your meal, e.g., at a restaurant, friend's, or family's house, then wait until the meal is in front of you before injecting any insulin. I have experienced hypoglycemia several times by not following this rule.

I must emphasize that the BID must be significantly reduced, by half or more, with the very first LCD/VLCD meal, to avoid hypoglycemia. Determining the correct BID will require some trial-and-error and you may find that the mathematical method for estimating your dosages presented at the end of this chapter is helpful.

Correction Bolus Insulin

A correction BID is given to correct high blood sugars with or between meals. Taking a correction dose within 5 hours of the last BID will result in insulin-stacking, which in turn, could cause hypoglycemia as a result of miscalculation or misestimation of subsequent BID. Therefore, it is prudent to avoid taking correction BID between meals when eating three meals/day. Rather, it is best to add or subtract a correction BID to the mealtime BID at each of the three meals/day. Taking a bedtime correction BID for an above-target blood sugar helps to keep basal insulin doses constant as explained above. If you are taking a BID for only one or two meals/day, then correction BID(s) can be taken as long as the previous dose was ≈ 5 hours earlier and the next dose will be ≈ 5 hours later. In other words, bolus insulin should not be given more often than ≈ 5 hours to prevent insulin-stacking, hypoglycemia, and the ability to accurately predict subsequent insulin doses. Although I understand the desire to quickly correct a high blood sugar, by following the strategies enumerated in this book, high blood sugars can be infrequent occurrences obviating the temptation to take between-meal correction BID.

Diluting Bolus Insulin

Smaller BID are required for those who make significant amounts of insulin in the 'honeymoon' phase of T1D and for children and adults following a LCD. Insulin pumps can deliver small BID, but U100 insulin pens can only deliver insulin in 1 IU increments and the smallest increment on an insulin syringe when using U100 insulin is 0.5 IU. Thus, if you want to administer insulin in increments of 0.1 IU, you will need to dilute your bolus insulin 5-fold and inject it with an insulin syringe. The manufacturer of the insulin you are using can provide you with the correct diluent. Both rapid-acting insulin analogs and short-acting regular insulin, when purchased in a 3-ml or 10-ml vial, can be diluted. Eli Lilly and Company kindly shipped lispro (Humalog) diluent to me at no cost.

The process of diluting insulin 5-fold that follows only applies to 10-ml vials of diluent. Once you obtain a 10-ml vial of diluent from the manufacturer, you need to use a 1 ml insulin syringe to withdraw 2 ml of the diluent from the 10-ml vial and discard it. Use of sterile technique is important so as not to contaminate your insulin with bacteria. When you remove diluent from the vial, it will create a vacuum in the vial. Use another insulin syringe with the plugger removed and insert it into the diluent vial with the vial upright on a table top to relieve the vacuum. Then take your insulin vial and withdraw 200 IU or 2 ml of insulin from the vial (2 withdrawals of 1 ml each) and inject it into the diluent vial. This process will create a vacuum in the insulin vial and a positive pressure inside the diluent vial, both of which can be relieved with the same syringe with plunger removed as before. This 5-fold dilution will dilute U-100 insulin to U-20 insulin, but other dilution ratios are possible if needed. Although this process is fairly straightforward, mistakes can be made. If you do not feel comfortable with diluting your own insulin, ask your pharmacist to do it for you. You will need to bring your insulin vial and the diluent vial to the pharmacy and tell the pharmacist what dilution ratio you prefer. They may charge you a fee for their services. Once the 5-fold dilution is complete, you will draw out 5 times more volume from the new diluted-insulin vial than you did previously. For example, if you need 1.3 IU of insulin, you will draw out an amount of diluted insulin that previously represented 6.5 IU (1.3 IU × 5).

Adjusting Bolus Insulin with Lifestyle Changes

There will be times when your lifestyle (diet, exercise, sleep, and/or travel) schedule will change either by choice or due to circumstances beyond your control. When changes are by choice, they should be small and gradual to allow time to adjust your BID, and if needed, to adjust your basal insulin dose as well. It is important to anticipate whether the lifestyle change is expected to increase or decrease your blood sugars so as to take precautions to avoid hypoglycemia. Lifestyle changes that would be expected to lower blood sugars should be anticipated and BID decreased empirically on day one. These lifestyle changes include decreasing carbohydrates when initiating a LCD, decreasing food intake for various reasons, or increasing exercise, e.g., participating or competing in a special sporting event. You should empirically reduce your insulin dose prior to these atypical meals or exercise sessions, monitor your blood glucose during exercise with a glucose meter or CGM, and have dextrose available to prevent or treat a low blood sugar.

Conversely, if you increase your dietary intake or reduce your exercise significantly, you would anticipate that your blood sugars will increase. In this situation, giving a higher insulin dose in anticipation of an increase in blood glucose is not a good idea because you can never be sure when or by how much your insulin requirements will increase. Although my insulin requirements typically increase on the day following an increase in dietary intake or reduction in exercise, I have experienced a lag period of 2–7 days before the blood glucose increases. It is safer to increase BID based on your actual blood glucose results. It may take a few days of adjusting BID to bring your blood sugars back to your target range depending on the degree and duration of the change in diet, exercise, or sleep, but your blood sugars will stabilize when your lifestyle stabilizes. This also applies to the changes in blood glucose that can occur with women's menstrual cycles or with an illness. It is better to respond to the actual increases in blood glucose than trying to anticipate when they might occur. When increasing BID to correct high blood sugars, do so conservatively, to avoid hypoglycemia.

Insulin Dosing in Children and Adolescents

When children do not eat their entire meal, choosing a BID is more challenging. If your child does not consistently eat his/her entire meal, the best approach is to postpone determining the dose and giving mealtime bolus insulin until after the meal is finished. The parent/caregiver can then assess the percentage of the meal eaten, using a kitchen scale or by eye, and adjust the BID accordingly. Adolescents with T1D may require more daily insulin per kg bodyweight compared to children or adults due to their accelerated growth. This increase in insulin requirements occurs gradually and may only be noticed in retrospect (see also, Dosing Basal Insulin, above).

Mathematical Estimation of Bolus Insulin Doses

Determining the BID inside a narrow therapeutic window that is 'just right' is, in my opinion, the most challenging problem that those with T1D have to solve in order to achieve normal blood sugars. My method of solving this problem, the inspiration for this book, starts with the LCD and adds timing and consistency of meals, exercise, and sleep to make insulin dose selection more predictable. Admittedly, keeping all these factors constant in order to have predictable BID does require a concerted effort. If we can manage to accomplish it, our insulin requirements will not vary much from day to day, but there will always be some variation in the blood glucose response to exogenous insulin for the reasons discussed in Chapter 3. You will be able to observe these day to day variations in the blood glucose response to identical doses of insulin, after identical meals, exercise, and sleep. Therefore, the goal will be to keep blood sugars in a range, in my case for example, 70–130 mg/dl (3.9–7.2 mM), rather than expecting the blood sugar to hit an exact target each and every time. There will also be times when life happens and our schedule, meals, exercise, or sleep change beyond our ability to prevent it. In this situation, the equations will not be as accurate, so don't expect that they will be.

I have experimented with numerous methods to estimate BID based on the blood glucose response to insulin doses on previous days. I will describe a method that is simple, effective, and self-adjusting to compensate for gradual changes in insulin requirements over time. This method requires that four conditions be met: 1) each given meal (or second best, the meal macronutrients) must remain constant from one day to the next, 2) that the basal insulin dose has remained constant for the past 2 days for NPH, 3 days for detemir (Levemir), 4 days for glargine (Lantus), and 5 days for degludec (Tresiba), before the effect of the basal insulin preparation stabilizes or in the case of insulin pump users, that the basal rate has been constant for the past 2 days and will remain constant 24-hours/day, everyday, 3) that insulin sensitivity does not change markedly from one day to the next due to changes in exercise, sleep, medications, time zones, etc., and 4) that bolus insulin is given no more frequently than about every 5 hours. Small changes in insulin sensitivity are expected and is one of the reasons blood glucose results change from day to day. A BID estimate (BIDE) can be calculated if these four conditions apply to your situation. If you do need to change the basal insulin dose or basal pump rate, do so, but keep in mind that the BIDE will not be as accurate over the next 2–5 days. The concept behind the calculation is simple. Bolus insulin serves two purposes, 1) to process the glucose, amino acids, and fatty acids that enter the bloodstream after a meal and to suppress liver glucose production which I will call meal insulin, MI, and 2) to adjust the pre-meal blood glucose (PreBG) up or down toward one's target blood glucose (TBG) which I will call correction insulin, CI. MI will be calculated retrospectively for every meal on previous days and represents the insulin dose that would be needed to process the meal without a change in blood glucose before and after the meal. Thus, BIDE = MI + CI, where MI is the previous day's MI, and CI = (PreBG − TBG) ÷ CF, where CF is the correction factor. The CI will be positive, i.e., give additional insulin, when the PreBG is greater than the TBG and negative, i.e., give less insulin, when the PreBG is less than the TBG. The CF represents an estimate of the increase (or decrease) in blood glucose per IU of insulin given (or withheld) and is always a positive number. The following equation can be used to estimate an initial value for CF: CF = 1,000 mg/dl ÷ TDID, where TDID is the total daily insulin dose or CF = 55.6 mM ÷ TDID. For example, for someone taking a total of 25 IU of insulin/day, CF = 1,000 mg/dl ÷ 25 IU = 40 mg/dl/IU or 55.6 mM ÷ 25 IU = 2.22 mM/IU. The CF is primarily a function of one's insulin sensitivity and bodyweight which is the rationale for using your TDID to calculate an initial estimate for CF. Thus, the CF that you use, will be customized to you and your blood glucose results. A different CF can be used for different meals and can be adjusted from the initial estimate over time to improve the BIDE. I started with a CF of 40 mg/dl/IU, and later decreased it to 35 mg/dl/IU to improve my results, but have not found using different CF values for different meals or bedtime to be helpful.

Decreasing CF from 40 mg/dl/IU to 35 mg/dl/IU results in giving less insulin for a low PreBG and more insulin for a high PreBG. Once the PostBG is measured, the meal insulin, MI, is calculated for each meal: MI = BID + ΔBG ÷ CF, where BID is the BID actually given, and ΔBG = Post BG − PreBG. When lifestyle changes occur that would be expected to lower blood sugars, the BIDE can be adjusted to give less insulin by increasing the TBG for each meal and at bedtime until your blood sugars return to normal. After I calculate the BIDE using the previous day's MI, I like to see what the predicted PostBG, PBG, would be if I used the MI from several days before. By simply rearranging the equation for BIDE and solving for TBG and substituting PBG for TBG, we get: PBG = PreBG + (MI − BIDE) × CF. This gives you the opportunity to revise your BIDE based on these PBG. I calculated values for 2-, 3-, and 4-day PBG in Table 5.4. Don't be alarmed by the results, I used a random number generator to determine all of the blood glucose results. The point of Table 5.4 is to show an example of the calculation results.

Using these equations is not required to achieve normal blood sugars. However, keeping a log similar to the one I use as shown in Table 5.4 is useful to be able to look back at previous BID and the ΔBG that resulted to determine your current insulin dose requirement. Using the equations gives me relief from 'decision fatigue' compared to 'experiential guessing' even though I know it is just an estimate. I do look back at the data from the previous several days and ask myself the question, 'In light of my previous responses to the insulin doses given, will this dose possibly cause hypoglycemia?' before making a final decision on the BID I actually inject. I would much prefer to err on the side of a mildly high blood glucose than on hypoglycemia. This applies particularly to the bedtime BID. If there is any time I would like to avoid hypoglycemia, it is while sleeping. As mentioned in Chapter 2, my monthly goal mean blood glucose is 98–104 mg/dl (5.4–5.8 mM) and SDBG 13.5–18 mg/dl (0.75–1.0 mM). These goals can be met as long as all, or almost all, of my blood glucose readings fall in the range 70–130 mg/dl (3.9–7.2 mM). As much as I would enjoy hitting my TBG 100% of the time, this is not necessary to achieve normal blood sugars. I actually confirmed this using 10,000 random numbers in the range 70–130 mg/dl (3.9–7.2 mM). The mean blood glucose was ≈ 100 mg/dl (≈ 5.6 mM) and SDBG was ≈ 18 mg/dl (≈ 1.0 mM).

I will also mention that since 2015, multiple smartphone apps have been developed to calculate/estimate BID. In the U.S., the FDA requires that these apps be reviewed for safety and accuracy before receiving FDA clearance. However, the majority of the apps available for download are not registered with the FDA. I have not used any of these apps myself.

Table 5.4 — Blood Glucose and Insulin Dose Log

Day	Time	BG mg/dl	BID IU	ΔBG mg/dl	MI IU	BIDE IU	2-day PBG	3-day PBG	4-day PBG
Sun	BRK	115	4.3	14	5.1	ND	ND	ND	ND
	LUN	129	3.2	-31	3.1	ND	ND	ND	ND
	DIN	98	2.5	-20	1.9	ND	ND	ND	ND
	BED	78	1.1	-4	0.4	ND	ND	ND	ND
Mon	BRK	74	4.4	16	4.1	4.4	ND	ND	ND
	LUN	90	2.9	-19	2.0	2.9	ND	ND	ND
	DIN	71	1.0	52	1.7	1.0	ND	ND	ND
	BED	123	1.0	-23	1.0	1.0	ND	ND	ND
Tues	BRK	100	4.1	-10	3.8	4.1	136	ND	ND
	LUN	90	1.7	-16	1.0	1.7	139	ND	ND

Master Type 1 Diabetes

	DIN	74	1.0	37	1.3	1.0	106	ND	ND
	BED	111	1.3	-10	1.4	1.3	77	ND	ND
Wed	BRK	101	3.8	1	3.9	3.8	110	146	ND
	LUN	102	1.1	-19	0.6	1.1	136	175	ND
	DIN	83	0.8	24	1.0	0.8	115	121	ND
	BED	107	1.6	-29	0.9	1.6	88	65	ND
Thur	BRK	78	3.3	2	2.7	3.3	97	107	143
	LUN	80	-0.0	35	0.4	-0.0	115	151	190
	DIN	115	1.4	9	2.1	1.4	110	125	131
	BED	124	1.6	-32	1.4	1.6	115	103	80
Fri	BRK	92	2.5	3	2.3	2.5	142	139	149
	LUN	95	0.3	22	0.8	0.3	105	120	156
	DIN	117	2.6	-25	2.4	2.6	61	71	86
	BED	92	1.2	-17	0.4	1.2	84	99	87
Sat	BRK	75	1.6	15	1.3	1.6	113	155	152
	LUN	90	0.5	6	0.4	0.5	88	93	108
	DIN	96	2.2	-11	1.8	2.2	91	52	62
	BED	85	0.0	-85		0.0	133	117	132

Note: ND = no data, CF = 35 mg/dl/IU, TBG = 100 mg/dl, BIDE = MI + (PreBG − TBG) ÷ CF, MI = BID + ΔBG ÷ CF, ΔBG = Post BG − PreBG, PBG = PreBG + (MI − BIDE) × CF, BRK = Breakfast, LUN = Lunch, DIN = Dinner, BED = Bedtime.

Insulin Pumps

Insulin pumps are designed to provide intensive insulin therapy by combining bolus and basal insulin infusions into one device. Insulin pumps have been in use for many years and the technology has progressively improved. This meta-analysis [Colquitt, J, et al., 2003] indicates that pump users prefer using rapid-acting insulin analogs and that lispro (Humalog) improved HbA1c by 0.26% compared to regular human insulin. When following a LCD, most will find that a rapid-acting insulin analog works best, but some may benefit from using short-acting regular insulin as discussed previously.

This study [Maiorino, MI, 2018] compared insulin pump therapy to multiple daily injections (MDI) in adults with T1D who had persistent HbA1c levels > 7.5% (58 mmol/mol). The 98 adults using insulin pump therapy had small, but statistically significant, improvements in glucose variability, fasting glycemia, and hypoglycemic events compared to the 125 adults using MDI. The HbA1c at the end of the 2-year follow-up period was the same in both groups: 8.1%. The SDBG was 58 mg/dl (3.2 mM) in the insulin pump group compared to 63 mg/dl (3.5 mM) in the MDI group. TDID was 0.63 IU/kg/day with pump therapy compared to 0.73 IU/kg/day with MDI. This large study [Karges, B, et al., 2017] compared glycemic control amongst 9,814 T1D patients using insulin pump therapy with 9,814 patients using MDI over a median of 3.7 years. Pump therapy was associated with lower rates of severe hypoglycemia and DKA compared to MDI. The average HbA1c was 8.04% with pump therapy compared to 8.22% with MDI. TDID was 0.84 IU/kg/day with pump therapy compared to 0.98 IU/kg/day with MDI.

From the viewpoint of both healthcare providers and insurance companies, insulin pumps are indicated for those with insulin-dependent diabetes who 1) cannot achieve goal blood sugar targets, 2) have frequent or serious hypoglycemic episodes, or 3) frequent hospital admissions for DKA with insulin injections. I have encountered many persons with T1D using insulin pumps who do not have any of these indications for their use. Many also use CGM to be discussed in Chapter 6. I have also encountered persons with T1D who switched from using an insulin pump to MDI after starting a LCD. There are many with T1D who do not use an insulin pump with, or without, a CGM for various reasons. Some, like me, prefer not to be attached to any device all the time as long as their glycemic management is satisfactory. Others are controlling their diabetes well enough that their insurance company will not cover the cost of an insulin pump or CGM and they cannot afford the device without the insurance covering most or all of the costs. Others do not have health insurance and cannot afford an insulin pump or CGM. For those without the option of using these devices, the strategies covered in this book can result in normal or near-normal blood sugars.

As with any technology, there are pros and cons to using an insulin pump. Advantages of an insulin pump include: 1) ability to adjust the basal insulin rate to compensate for unplanned or prolonged exercise, 2) elimination of the need for MDI, 3) ability to accurately deliver insulin in 0.1 unit increments eliminating the need to dilute insulin, 4) when combined with a CGM, the low-glucose warnings and insulin-suspension feature, may prevent harm from hypoglycemia, and 5) in studies, small improvements in some measures of glycemic control have been demonstrated which might translate when using a LCD. Disadvantages of an insulin pump include: 1) cost of the pump and supplies, 2) pump failure or infusion set problems causing DKA if not recognized in time, 3) insulin infusion set infections, hypersensitivity, and technical problems [Heinemann, L, et al., 2012], and 4) lipodystrophy — damage to the fatty layer under the skin — can occur if infusion sites are overused, i.e., not rotated properly, and 5) the need to continuously monitor and care for an attached device.

Without an RCT in those utilizing a LCD and the other strategies in this book, it is difficult to know if an insulin pump with, or without, a CGM would result in improvements above and beyond MDI and SMBG. Until such studies can demonstrate superiority of one over another as a guide, I think each individual needs to make their own decision about whether or not to use an insulin pump and/or CGM assuming they can afford the financial costs involved. Insulin pumps can be used with the strategies in this book including the BIDE prediction equations by keeping the basal insulin rate constant 24 hours/day and not allowing the pump to calculate the BID based on carbohydrate intake. Taking advantage of the insulin-suspend feature, especially at night, is a good idea for one's safety.

The Artificial Pancreas

The artificial pancreas or hybrid closed-loop system combines an insulin pump, CGM, and software to control the rate of insulin delivery per the IG readings of the CGM and user settings. In 2016 the United States Food & Drug Administration (FDA) approved the first artificial pancreas, the Medtronic's MiniMed 670G System. In a 6-month clinical trial [Brown, SA, et al., 2019], 112 with T1D were randomized to the artificial pancreas and 56 were randomized to a sensor-augmented insulin pump (control group). After 6 months, the HbA1c in the control group decreased from 7.40% at baseline to 7.39% and the HbA1c in the artificial pancreas group decreased from 7.40% at baseline to 7.06% (− 0.34%). A similar clinical trial [Tauschmann, M, et al., 2018] compared the effectiveness of an artificial pancreas with an insulin pump/CGM (control group) in persons with T1D, aged 6 years and older. Participants in both study groups used a modified 640G insulin pump, Enlite 3 glucose sensor (Medtronic), and Contour Next Link 2.4 glucose meter. The study specifically sought to include patients with suboptimal diabetes control with HbA1c values between 7.5% and 10%. The HbA1c in the artificial pancreas group was reduced from 8.0% to 7.4% after the 12-week intervention period. The HbA1c in control group decreased from 7.8% to 7.7%. Time spent with hypoglycemia was less in the artificial pancreas group (2.6% of time) compared to the control group (3.9% of time). The average increase in bodyweight in the artificial pancreas group was 2.2 kg compared to 1.4 kg in the control group. It is a common finding in studies that improving glycemic control with additional insulin while on a LFHCD increases bodyweight. This meta-analysis [Bekiari, E, et al., 2018] of artificial pancreas treatment for outpatients with T1D found improvements in proportion of time in the near-normoglycemic range (3.9–10.0 mM (70–180 mg/dl)) over a 24-hour period, weighted mean difference of 9.62% and relative reduction of mean blood glucose levels by 0.48 mM (8.6 mg/dl), which was consistent with the HbA1c reduction of about 0.3% recorded in trials with a duration of more than eight weeks per intervention compared to the baseline values that ranged from 6.9% to 8.6%. No difference between artificial pancreas use and control treatment was seen in the mean TDID (− 0.21 IU).

In December 2019, the FDA approved the t:slim X2 Pump linked with the Dexcom G6 CGM. The t:slim X2™ insulin pump with Control-IQ™ technology is an artificial pancreas designed to help increase time in range, 70–180 mg/dl (3.9–10.0 mM), using Dexcom G6 CGM values to predict glucose levels 30 minutes ahead. Based on those predictions, it adjusts insulin delivery rate accordingly, which includes delivery of automatic correction boluses as often as hourly https://www.tandemdiabetes.com.

Features include:
- Delivers an automatic correction bolus if sensor glucose is predicted to be above 180 mg/dl (10.0 mM).
- Increases basal insulin delivery if sensor glucose is predicted to be above 160 mg/dl (8.9 mM).
- Maintains active Personal Profile settings.
- Decreases basal insulin delivery if sensor glucose is predicted to be below 112.5 mg/dl (6.3 mM).
- Stops basal insulin delivery if sensor glucose is predicted to be below 70 mg/dl (3.9 mM)."

The Control-IQ™ technology has an optional 'sleep activity' mode that allows the basal range to be adjusted to seek a target glucose in the range 110–120 mg/dl (6.1–6.7 mM). This optional setting does not allow any auto-correction boluses while it is activated. It would be helpful to have a RCT in those with T1D following the LCD and the strategies discussed in this book compared those using: 1) MDI and SMBG, 2) an insulin pump/CGM, and 3) an artificial pancreas set to seek a normal target blood glucose.

In Table 5.3, I compare several metrics from the study groups above with my personal results using MDI, SMBG four times/day, and the other strategies detailed in this book.

Table 5.3 — Comparison of Metrics of Glucose Control

Parameter	Artificial pancreas group (n=46)	Insulin pump/ CGM group (n=40)	Dr. Runyan's monthly results (n=1)
Average Blood Glucose	160 mg/dl 8.9 mM	175 mg/dl 9.7 mM	≈ 100 mg/dl ≈ 5.6 mM
Standard Deviation of Blood Glucose	63 mg/dl 3.5 mM	68 mg/dl 3.8 mM	≈ 18 mg/dl ≈ 1.00 mM
Total Daily Insulin Dose	0.81 IU/kg/day	0.71 IU/kg/day	≈ 0.34 IU/kg/day

Reference: [Tauschmann, M, et al., 2018]

While a LCD/VLCD with consistent meals, exercise, and sleep may improve or normalize blood sugars when combined with an artificial pancreas, the equations I presented above to calculate BIDE cannot be used with an artificial pancreas device which automatically adjusts the basal insulin rate and/or gives bolus insulin doses as frequently as hourly.

Dana M. Lewis offers a free DIY guide on automated insulin delivery at https://www.artificialpancreasbook.com/download and there are other DIY algorithms available online. I have no personal experience using these algorithms.

6 – Tests and Devices to Measure Glucose

"Learn as if you have to learn forever, live as if you die tomorrow."
Elliott P. Joslin, MD, America's first diabetologist.

Hemoglobin A1c

Hemoglobin A1c (HbA1c), as you probably know, is a laboratory test your physician orders several times a year to monitor your blood sugar control. HbA1c is formed when glucose binds to a hemoglobin molecule. Hemoglobin is the protein in red blood cells that carries oxygen from the lungs to all the tissues in the body. Red blood cells are made in the bone marrow and circulate in the bloodstream for about 100–120 days. During this time, glucose binds with hemoglobin in proportion to its concentration in the blood. The higher the HbA1c, the higher the blood glucose was during the time the hemoglobin was in circulation. HbA1c was identified in 1958, but its elevation in persons with diabetes was first recognized in 1969. HbA1c became a routine medical laboratory test in 1977 and was the primary means to monitor a patient's glycemic control since home glucose meters were just becoming available at that time. Since many patients either do not have, or do not use, their home glucose meters, healthcare providers still rely on the HbA1c result as a surrogate for average blood glucose. But you should understand the limitations of the HbA1c test. The HbA1c result is influenced by other factors in addition to the average blood glucose in the previous 2–3 months. This is important because healthcare providers often rely on this test to make adjustments to your treatment regimen. These factors include any condition that alters the red blood cell lifespan, e.g., hemolytic anemia, iron-deficiency anemia, kidney failure, hemoglobinopathies (sickle cell disease and thalassemia), or recent red blood cell transfusions or donations [Dijkstra, A, et al., 2017]. Race and age also affect the HbA1c result [Little, RR, et al., 2009]. Still other unknown factors cause a 'glycation gap' between HbA1c and self-monitored blood glucose (SMBG). This has lead to a hypothesis that genetic differences exist between individuals causing some to be 'low glycators' and others to be 'high glycators' [Snieder, H, et al., 2001]. This study [Khera, PK, et al., 2008] measured the glucose concentration inside (exposed to hemoglobin) and outside (blood glucose) the red blood cells (RBC) of 5 nondiabetic, 10 T1D, and 11 T2D subjects to test the hypothesis that differences between the two might explain the 'glycation gap' observed with HbA1c. The authors were able to conclude that "… we have identified a variable in the RBC — the trans-membrane glucose gradient — that is a strong candidate to introduce interindividual variability into the rate of HbA1c formation." This means the glucose concentration inside the RBC is lower than outside in low glycators resulting in lower HbA1c values than the mean blood glucose would predict. The opposite would occur in high glycator's, i.e., HbA1c is higher than would be predicted by the mean blood glucose. Thus, it is important to know that HbA1c is not simply of measure of mean blood glucose and an individual's mean blood glucose can't necessarily be inferred from their HbA1c. See my blog post #23 for additional information

https://ketogenicdiabeticathlete.wordpress.com/2016/04/23/23-the-hba1c-test-does-it-just-reflect-average-blood-glucose/. Given these limitations of HbA1c, I decided to stop measuring my HbA1c in 2015.

This study [Nathan, DM, et al, 2008] took data from the Diabetes Control and Complications Trial (DCCT) to determine the correlation between average blood glucose and HbA1c. The linear regression equations were as follows: average glucose (mg/dl) = 28.7 × HbA1c (%) −

46.7 or average glucose (mM) = 1.59 × HbA1c (%) − 2.59 (R^2 = 0.84). An earlier study [Rohlfing, CL, et al., 2002] using data from the DCCT gave similar results. These equations are used on lab reports to provide a rough estimate of average blood glucose from the measured HbA1c. Interestingly, if this equation is used to estimate the HbA1c from the participants following a VLCD whose mean blood glucose was 106 mg/dl (5.9 mM) in the online survey [Lennerz, BS, et al., 2018] mentioned in Chapter 4, the HbA1c is 5.32% which is quite different that the actual mean HbA1c of 5.67%. There are many potential explanations for this difference, but suffice it to say that HbA1c is just a rough estimate of mean glycemia.

Since June 2011, the preferred unit of measure for HbA1c was changed from percentage to mmols/mol in many countries. When HbA1c is reported as a percentage, it is called the DCCT (Diabetes Control and Complications Trial) unit, whereas, when reported as mmols/mol, it is known as the IFCC (International Federation of Clinical Chemistry) unit. To convert HbA1c (%) to HbA1c (mmols/mol), multiply by 6.22. To convert HbA1c (mmols/mol) to HbA1c (%), divide by 6.22.

The bottomline is that no one measure of blood glucose is perfect. If your HbA1c does not correlate with your mean blood glucose by SMBG or mean IG by CGM, possible reasons include 1) the factors mentioned above for deviations of HbA1c from the mean blood glucose, 2) infrequent measurements of blood glucose by SMBG, 3) an inaccurate home glucose meter, or 4) an inaccurate CGM device. Measuring fructosamine or glycated albumin might help determine the source of discrepancy. In general, treatment decisions should be based on SMBG and/or CGM data from an accurate device rather than HbA1c, fructosamine, and glycated albumin results. Equally important, since HbA1c, fructosamine, and glycated albumin are measures of average blood glucose, they provide no information about the variability of blood glucose. A person with frequent low and high blood sugars could have a reasonable HbA1c result, but still be at risk for both long-term diabetic complications and death from hypoglycemia. This is why I advocate tracking both average blood glucose and glycemic variability using the SDBG of SMBG or SDIG of CGM. Those with T1D should be seeking normal glycemia and glycemic variability with minimal hypoglycemia.

Fructosamine and Glycated Albumin

Glycated albumin is a laboratory test that measures the binding of glucose to serum albumin as a measure of average blood glucose in the previous 2–4 weeks. Serum albumin is the most abundant protein ($\approx$ 60–70%) in the blood. Fructosamine is similar to glycated albumin, but also measures glycated lipoproteins, globulins, and immunoglobulins, in particular, IgA. In this study [Selvin, E, et al., 2014], elevated levels of fructosamine and glycated albumin were positively associated with development of diabetes and its microvascular complications (diabetic retinopathy and nephropathy) during two decades of follow-up with a prognostic value comparable to that of HbA1c. Fructosamine and glycated albumin are more representative of average blood sugar than HbA1c when short-term assessment of blood sugar control is needed, e.g., during pregnancy or when assessing the effectiveness of a new therapy including diet, lifestyle, or medication. And as mentioned previously, fructosamine and glycated albumin can help determine the cause of a discrepancy between HbA1c and average SMBG and/or CGM measurements [Danese, E, et al., 2015].

Home Blood Glucose Meters

The home blood glucose meter is a valuable tool for persons with diabetes to get immediate feedback on the effect of diet, exercise, and medications on their blood sugar levels. Prior to this development, those with diabetes could only measure glucose in their urine which usually did not register as present until after the blood glucose exceeded 170 mg/dl (9.44 mM). Thus, it was impossible to achieve anywhere close to normal blood sugars. Home blood glucose meters began to be developed and sold in the 1970s and have improved in many respects since then. Today, home blood glucose meters are small, lightweight, inexpensive, easy to use, and rapidly provide a result with a tiny drop of blood [Clarke, SF, et al., 2012]. The accuracy of your blood glucose meter is of paramount importance when seeking normal blood sugars. This study [Klonoff, DC, et al., 2018] conducted in the U.S., compared the accuracy of 18 home glucose meters which represented ≈ 90% of the commercially available systems used from 2013 to 2015. The top five most accurate blood glucose meters were 1) Contour Next, 2) Accu-Check Aviva Plus, 3) Walmart ReliOn Confirm (Micro), 4) CVS Advanced, and 5) Freestyle Freedom Lite. Another study [Ekhlaspour, L, et al., 2017] also conducted in the U.S., compared the accuracy of 17 commercially available glucose meters. The top five most accurate blood glucose meters were 1) Contour Next, 2) StatStrip Xpress, 3) OneTouch VerioIQ, 4) Accu-Chek Nano, and 5) Freestyle Freedom Lite. I suggest using one of these accurate meters a minimum of four times daily as a tool to achieve normal blood sugars (unless you have an accurate CGM device). Follow the directions for use that comes with your meter and clean your hands before measuring your blood glucose. Using the lancet device that comes with the meter on the side of the distal third of your fingers is more comfortable than on the pad of the finger where most of the sensory nerve endings are located. The depth the lancet extends into the skin is adjustable as is the pressure you apply to your finger. With practice, you can learn how much pressure will yield an adequate size drop of blood for your meter, thus minimizing trauma to the skin. Occasionally, a defective blood glucose strip will give a spurious result without an error code being displayed on the meter. If you suspect the blood glucose reading may be in error, simply repeat it with a new strip. Finally, blood glucose readings can become erroneous as a home blood glucose meter ages. Many years ago, over a 4-month period, I experienced numerous hypoglycemic episodes from a 2-year old meter that started giving falsely-high blood glucose results causing me to overdose on insulin. During this period, I felt that I came close to dying from several nocturnal hypoglycemic episodes. The lessons I learned were: get the most accurate blood glucose meter available, that technology is fallible, and when things aren't going well, question everything!

Using a Glucose Meter to Normalize Blood Sugars

If you have an accurate CGM, some of the suggestions that follow may not apply to you while using your CGM. Consistently using an accurate home blood glucose meter at least four times daily is necessary to achieve normal blood sugars with T1D. If you are eating three evenly-spaced meals daily, I suggest measuring blood sugar on arising in the morning (fasting blood sugar) which usually coincides with breakfast, before lunch, before dinner, and at bedtime. If you only eat one or two meals daily, you should still check your blood sugar four times daily. This gives you the opportunity to take a correction BID if your blood sugar is above target, or to take dextrose if your blood sugar is below target. There are additional times when blood sugar should be measured. These times include 1) if you do not feel right (may be a symptom of hypoglycemia), 2) before and while operating a vehicle, 3) before and after a new or quite different exercise session and during an unusually long exercise session, 4) before taking any insulin or medication that would lower blood sugar, and 5) ≈ 2–3 hours after a meal if you have been experiencing hypoglycemia after meals to detect impending hypoglycemia. Some of these times may coincide with the pre-meal and bedtime blood sugar checks. Measuring blood glucose only occasionally and/or not taking appropriate action based on the results are behaviors typical of those with poorly-controlled T1D. I also suggest doing a blood glucose profile periodically by checking blood sugar eight times in one day if you do not use a CGM. The additional four blood sugar checks can be done evenly-spaced between your usual four checks. This will reveal any unexpected high or low blood sugars between the usual blood sugar checks. A blood glucose profile can be done as frequently as needed to help you and your physician adjust your insulin, diet, and exercise regimen.

To calculate SDBG you use can use a spreadsheet on your home computer (excel for windows or numbers for mac) or you can use this free online calculator at https://www.calculator.net/standard-deviation-calculator.html. The software that comes with some home blood glucose meters, e.g., Contour Next, https://glucofacts.ascensia.com/GFD/en-us, calculates mean blood glucose and SDBG for you. Data from many different home glucose and ketone meters, CGM devices, and insulin pumps can be uploaded and analyzed for free at https://www.tidepool.org/users/devices.

Continuous Glucose Monitors

Continuous glucose monitors (CGM) have been in use for more than decade. They measure the interstitial glucose (IG) concentration which is close to the actual blood glucose concentration but delayed by ≈ 15 mins. Most CGM have a sensor inserted by the user on the abdomen or arm. The accuracy of CGM have improved over the years and many important features have been added. CGM sensors relay the readings, usually every five minutes, to a receiver, an insulin pump, or a smartphone. Some models can send IG results immediately to a second person's smartphone — perhaps a parent, partner, or caregiver. Analysis of the data from these devices can assess how close you are to meeting your goals and to identify areas for further improvement. CGM also have alarms to alert you to low or high IG readings or that you are quickly approaching a low or high IG reading based on the rate of change of the IG reading. This is especially useful when sleeping, driving a vehicle, or exercising. Some CGM devices require blood glucose to be measured 2–4 times a day for the purpose of calibrating the CGM. Some newer models do not require any calibration, e.g., Dexcom G6 and the Freestyle Libre 2. Insulin pumps can be connected to some CGM and programmed to suspend the insulin infusion for a low IG reading, while others, can adjust the rate of insulin delivery forming an 'artificial pancreas' or hybrid closed-loop system which was discussed in Chapter 5. Since the features of CGM vary and change with time, you will need to research each of the available CGM and pick the specific device that suits your needs.

The Guardian™ Sensor 3 from Medtronic can be used as part of the Minimed 670G as an artificial pancreas device, with the Minimed 630G insulin pump to suspend the insulin infusion for low glucose readings, or as a stand-alone CGM device https://www.medtronicdiabetes.com. The Guardian™ Sensor 3 sensor needs to be replaced every 7 days. The Guardian™ Sensor 3 requires finger-stick blood glucose calibrations twice daily.

The Dexcom G6® CGM sensor is replaced every 10 days, does not require finger-stick blood glucose calibration, and can work with the Tandem t:slim X2 with Basal-IQ Technology as discussed in Chapter 5 at https://www.dexcom.com.

The Freestyle Libre 2 CGM made by Abbott at https://www.freestylelibre.us/system-overview/freestyle-libre-2.html transmits IG readings to a reader (or smartphone) only when the reader is placed in close proximity to the sensor on the body, but has the added feature of optional, real-time, glucose alarms that notify you if your blood glucose is below or above your set limits as long as the reader or smartphone is within 20 feet of the sensor. As long as you take a reading every eight hours, it will acquire an IG reading every five minutes and the data can be uploaded to your computer or smartphone and analyzed with software. The sensor is replaced every 14 days. The Freestyle Libre 2 CGM does not require finger-stick blood glucose calibration. The mean absolute relative difference (MARD) was found to be 9.2% for adults and 9.7% for children. MARD is a measure of CGM accuracy, the lower the number, the better the accuracy.

When comparing the accuracy of different devices it is important to note the date of the study since CGM continue to improve over time. The accuracy of CGM can be assessed by comparison to SMBG, laboratory measured glucose, head-to-head trials of two different CGM devices, or outcome trials looking for improvements in HbA1c and reduction in the number and duration of hypoglycemic episodes [Bailey, TS, 2017]. This small study [Biagi, L, et al., 2018] with one female and five male subjects with T1D measured the accuracy of the Medtronic Paradigm Enlite-2 CGM, under closed-loop therapy, worn by each subject before, during, and after exercise. Accuracy of the CGM as measured by MARD with plasma glucose measurements showed a degradation of accuracy caused by the onset of aerobic exercise (cycle-ergometer) not seen with anaerobic exercise (weightlifting). This study [Taleb, N, et al., 2016] also found a lower accuracy during exercise for both the Dexcom G4 Platinum and Medtronic Paradigm Veo Enlite system. This study [Moser, O, et al., 2016] found the accuracy of the Medtronic Enlite, Guardian® REAL-Time CGM to be acceptable during several levels of intensity of continuous and intermittent exercise except during continuous high-intensity exercise. This study [Bally, L, et al., 2016] found the accuracy of the Dexcom G4 Platinum CGM system to be acceptable during intermittent high-intensity and continuous moderate-intensity exercise.

In this study [Heinemann, L, et al., 2018], the benefits of using a CGM included a reduction in HbA1c from 7.6% to 7.4% (−0.2%) and a reduction in hypoglycemic episodes especially in those with a history of hypoglycemic unawareness or severe hypoglycemia: defined as requiring assistance or hospitalization. This study [Lind, M, et al., 2017] showed a similar reduction in HbA1c from 8.35% to 7.92% (−0.43%) and a reduction in hypoglycemic episodes. It is difficult to extrapolate the results of these clinical trials to those seeking normal blood sugars using the strategies in this book. Simply trying out and assessing the value of a CGM for yourself is probably the best option. If you measure your blood glucose four times daily with an accurate meter, you can calculate the MARD of your CGM device for yourself using the formula in this paper [Reiterer, F, et al., 2017]. For those who can't afford to purchase a CGM, I think it is safe to say, at least from my experience, that normal blood sugars can be achieved safely without a CGM device. To date, I have made a personal decision not to use a CGM. There are four reasons for this decision: 1) I feel more 'normal' not having a device attached to my body all the time, 2) I don't want to have to worry about damaging the device while exercising, swimming, scuba diving, etc., and 3) hypoglycemia is a rare event now and I feel safe not wearing a CGM to detect hypoglycemia. A CGM would have been useful to me at certain times in the past, but now that hypoglycemia is a rare event, I no longer feel my glycemic control would be much improved with the use of a CGM. Were I to resume doing prolonged exercise, like triathlons, I would use the Freestyle Libre 2. Please don't let my reasons for not using a CGM have any bearing on your decision-making process. When it comes to treating your T1D, you should always do what is best for you. "CGM should be considered in all children and adolescents with T1D, whether using injections or insulin pump infusion, as an additional tool to help improve glucose control" [Riddle, MC, et al., 2020, S163–S182.].

7 – Formulating an Exercise Regimen

"Exercise is king, nutrition is queen, put them together and you have a kingdom."
Jack LaLanne, The First Nationally Recognized Fitness Guru.

"Exercise is the surest and best intervention we have to increase health-span and lifespan."
Dr. Eric Verdin, President and CEO, Buck Institute for Research on Aging.

"Weakness is never a strength. Strength is never a weakness."
Mark Bell, Powerlifter, Entrepreneur.

"It is better to discuss how far you have walked, than how little you have eaten."
Elliott P. Joslin, MD, America's first diabetologist.

Exercise for Health and Longevity

Prior to beginning any exercise program, it is prudent to get clearance from your physician regarding the particular exercises you would like to pursue due the increased risk for CVD and to make accommodations for any long-term diabetic complications you may have, if any. You may need to be screened for coronary artery disease as directed by your physician. If you have diabetic complications, you may need to avoid certain exercises until such time that your complications heal. For example, long-distance running with peripheral neuropathy can cause unnecessary foot injuries and are completely avoidable with a different choice of exercise, e.g., swimming. Similarly, if proliferative diabetic retinopathy or severe non-proliferative diabetic retinopathy is present, then vigorous-intensity aerobic or resistance exercise may be contraindicated because of the risk of triggering vitreous hemorrhage or retinal detachment [Riddle, MC, et al., 2020]. Consultation with an ophthalmologist before engaging in an intense exercise regimen may be appropriate. It is also prudent to get your blood sugars under reasonably good control before adding exercise to your lifestyle. Initiating a new exercise with a low (< 100 mg/dl (< 5.6 mM)) or high (> 200 mg/dl (> 11.1 mM)) blood sugar is not a good idea since, depending on the type of exercise, your blood sugar could go from low to lower, or from high to higher. If you are new to exercise, you should start with easy exercise of short duration and gradually increase the intensity and/or duration over time, both for your body's sake and so that you can understand your blood sugar response to the activity.

In the United States, nearly $117 billion in annual health care costs and 10% of all premature deaths are associated with failure to meet the recommended levels of physical activity. Only 26% of men, 19% of women, and 20% of adolescents meet the physical activity guideline recommendations, despite the fact that most individuals in the U.S. are able to meet the minimum recommendations. As we age, our physical capability, strength, and muscle mass will have a direct impact on both our health-span and lifespan. This study [Wang, H, et al., 2019] of nonagenarians in China found that muscle mass predicts mortality in women and points out that in other studies, physical disability, mobility limitation, cognitive impairment, and poor physical performance, are associated with increased mortality. The majority of those with T1D also do not meet the physical activity guidelines. Certainly, hypoglycemia represents a significant barrier to regular exercise participation [Colberg,

SR, et al., 2015]. With the strategies discussed in this book, you will find that hypoglycemia can, indeed, be a rare event with a well-planned exercise and insulin-dosing program.

The following are some important points from the 2018 Physical Activity Guidelines for Americans regarding the health benefits of exercise and exercise guidelines for children, adolescents, adults, and older adults including those with T1D [2018 Physical Activity Guidelines Advisory Committee, 2nd edition, 2018].

1. Everyone should engage in regular physical activity to improve overall health and fitness and to prevent negative health outcomes.
2. The benefits of physical activity occur in generally healthy people of all ages, in people at risk of developing chronic diseases, and in people with chronic conditions (including T1D) or disabilities.
3. One consistent finding from research studies is that once the health benefits from physical activity begin to accumulate, additional amounts of activity provide additional benefits. Therefore, the amount, intensity, or types of exercise should be gradually increased over time as tolerated.
4. Some benefits of physical activity can be achieved immediately, such as reduced blood pressure and feelings of anxiety, improvements in sleep and insulin sensitivity, and some aspects of cognitive function. Other benefits, such as increased cardiorespiratory fitness, increased muscular size and strength, decreases in depressive symptoms, and sustained reduction in blood pressure, require a few weeks or months of participation in physical activity.
5. The benefits of physical activity also outweigh the risk of injury and heart attacks, two concerns that may prevent people from becoming physically active.

6. Both aerobic and muscle-strengthening physical activity lower blood pressure in persons with hypertension (high blood pressure).

7. Exercise strengthens bones, joints, and muscles which are critical to the ability to do daily activities without physical limitations such as climbing stairs, working in the garden, or carrying a small child.

8. Progressive muscle-strengthening activities preserve or increase muscle mass, strength, and power. Improvements occur in children and adolescents as well as in younger and older adults. Though aerobic activity does not increase muscle mass in the same way that muscle-strengthening activity does, it can help slow the loss of muscle with aging.

9. Adults should move more and sit less throughout the day. Some physical activity is better than none. Adults who sit less and do any amount of moderate-to-vigorous physical activity gain some health benefits.

10. For substantial health benefits, adults should do at least 150–300 mins per week of moderate-intensity, or 75–150 mins per week of vigorous-intensity aerobic activity, or an equivalent combination of both. Aerobic activity should preferably be spread throughout the week.

11. Additional health benefits are gained by engaging in physical activity beyond the equivalent of 300 mins of moderate-intensity physical activity per week.

12. Adults should also do muscle-strengthening activities of moderate or greater intensity that involves all major muscle groups on 2 or more days per week, as these activities provide additional health benefits.

13. As part of their weekly physical activity, older adults should do multicomponent physical activity that includes balance training as well as aerobic and muscle-strengthening activities.

14. Older adults should determine their level of effort for physical activity relative to their level of fitness.
15. Older adults with chronic conditions should understand whether and how their conditions affect their ability to do regular physical activity safely.
16. When older adults cannot do 150 mins of moderate-intensity aerobic activity per week because of chronic conditions, they should be as physically active as their abilities and conditions allow.

Table 7.1 lists numerous health benefits of exercise which I hope will inspire you to pursue some type of physical activity on a daily basis.

Table 7.1 — Health Benefits Associated With Regular Physical Activity
Children and Adolescents
1. Improved bone health and weight status (ages 3 through 17 years)
2. Improved muscular fitness and cardiometabolic health (ages 6 through 17 years)
3. Improved cognition and reduced risk of depression (ages 6 to 13 years)

Adults and Older Adults
1. Lower risk of all-cause mortality
2. Lower risk of CVD and mortality
3. Lower risk of hypertension (high blood pressure)
4. Lower risk of type 2 diabetes (due to improved insulin sensitivity)
5. Lower risk of abnormal blood lipid profile
6. Lower risk of cancers of the bladder, breast, colon, endometrium, esophagus, kidney, lung, and stomach
7. Improved cognition and reduced risk of dementia (including Alzheimer's disease)
8. Improved quality of life, sleep, and reduced anxiety and depression

9. Slowed and reduced weight gain
10. Weight loss, particularly when combined with reduced calorie intake
11. Prevention of weight regain following initial weight loss
12. Increased muscle mass which burns more calories even while resting and sleeping
13. Improved bone health and physical function
14. Lower risk of falls and fall-related injuries in older adults

Note: The information in this table was taken from Table 2–1 in [2018 Physical Activity Guidelines Advisory Committee, 2nd edition, 2018].

Aerobic Exercise

Aerobic exercise involves continuous body movement over varying lengths of time which trains both skeletal muscle and the cardiopulmonary systems. Examples of aerobic exercise include walking, running, bicycling, rowing, swimming, and many more. The word 'aerobic' means that oxygen is utilized in the burning of glucose and fat to generate adenosine triphosphate (ATP): the universal source of cellular energy in humans and animals. This is in contrast to 'anaerobic,' in which oxygen is not involved in making ATP from glucose by its conversion to lactate. As the intensity of aerobic exercise increases, an increasing proportion of ATP is generated anaerobically as a result of the inability of aerobic oxidation of glucose and fat to keep pace with the rate of ATP utilization. Regular aerobic physical activity is without doubt beneficial for maintaining muscle mass and improving cardiopulmonary fitness, body composition, and insulin sensitivity. Adoption of a LCD/VLCD may be advantageous for endurance athletes by facilitating a 2-fold increase in fat oxidation during exercise [Volek, JS, et al., 2016].

Resistance Exercise

Resistance exercise involves pushing or pulling against a weight, band, or bodyweight and is a key physical activity that is necessary for an optimal health-span and lifespan. Examples of resistance exercise include lifting and carrying weights, use of elastic bands, and bodyweight exercises. This review article [McCarthy, O, et al., 2019] on the role of resistance exercise in those with T1D concluded that "Perhaps most importantly, the wider metabolic, vascular, and respiratory roles of skeletal muscle each have particular relevance for individuals with T1D, whom are predisposed to greater pathological risk within these systems by virtue of the condition. Thus, the positive, adaptive health benefits associated with the hypertrophic and strength benefits accompanied with resistance exercise should be promoted as a necessary adjunct to standard diabetes care."

Resistance exercise improves body composition and strength of muscle and bone making us more resistant to falling and suffering life-threatening injuries, like hip fracture and head trauma, as we age. Resistance training improves strength and increases muscle size by gradually increasing the amount of weight (intensity), and/or number of reps/sets (volume) lifted over time. Our bodies respond to gradual and progressive increases in resistance exercise by adapting to the stress applied. This adaptation involves an increase in muscle size, strength, and neural innervation to recruit more muscle fibers during contractions. As muscle size increases, it becomes a large sink for glucose disposal, improves insulin sensitivity, and decreases exogenous insulin doses in those with T1D. Over time, one will inevitably need to reduce the rate of increase in intensity and may need to decrease the volume (# sets/reps) in order to continue increasing the intensity (weight). Another objective is to limit injuries by making increases in both intensity and volume gradually. I have had many sprains, strains, and overuse injuries due to excessive increases in intensity/volume. I hope I have learned my lesson at this point.

This study [Yardley, JE, et al., 2013] compared the acute effects of 45 mins of aerobic vs. resistance exercise in 12 physically active individuals with type 1 diabetes on glycemia. "Plasma glucose decreased from 8.4 to 6.8 mM (151 to 122 mg/dl) during resistance exercise and from 9.2 to 5.8 mM (166 to 104 mg/dl) during aerobic exercise. During recovery, glucose levels did not change significantly after resistance exercise, but increased by 2.2 mM (40 mg/dl) after aerobic exercise. Resistance exercise causes less initial decline in blood glucose during the activity, but is associated with more prolonged reductions in post-exercise glycemia than aerobic exercise. This might account for HbA1c reductions found in studies of resistance exercise, but not aerobic exercise in T1D."

High Intensity Interval Training

HIIT exercise involves short periods of very intense exertion alternating with short periods of rest. HIIT can be aerobic, resistance, or involve both types of activity. Short sprints followed by short rest periods is an example of aerobic HIIT while using near-maximal resistance exercises with short rest periods in-between is an example of resistance HIIT. This study [Cipryan, L, et al., 2018] found that adoption of a VLCD over 4 weeks increased the rate of maximal fat oxidation and did not adversely affect either time to exhaustion during graded exercise tests or cardiorespiratory responses to HIIT compared with the subjects usual Western diet. HIIT exercise is a time-efficient form of exercise that improves insulin sensitivity, promotes body fat loss [Viana, RB, et al., 2019], and improves muscle strength and size. When HIIT is done twice weekly, as is often suggested, insulin sensitivity will vary from day to day making blood sugar management quite difficult. However, HIIT exercise can be modified and done on a daily basis by using fewer muscle groups each day and rotating through different muscle groups on different days. This tends to stabilize one's insulin sensitivity and blood sugars while still allowing muscular recovery. Aerobic HIIT can be done daily by reducing the volume (# sets/reps) of activity so that one can recover by the following day.

Exercise Training Improves Insulin Sensitivity

Exercise improves insulin sensitivity and the ability of muscle tissue to take up glucose both acutely (after a single exercise session) and chronically (with regular exercise training). "A single bout of moderate intensity exercise can increase glucose uptake by at least 40%. The combination of aerobic exercise training and resistance exercise training may be more effective than either exercise mode alone. Aerobic exercise may increase insulin sensitivity without a measurable increase in VO_2 max or VO_2 peak. A dose effect may be evident, with greater exercise volumes and higher exercise intensities, including HIIT or sprint interval training, producing greater benefits to insulin sensitivity" [Bird, SR, 2017]. In this study [Koivisto, VA, et al., 1986], the TDID decreased by 6% from reductions in lunch and dinner BID on exercise days consistent with improved insulin sensitivity.

Exercise prevents and treats insulin resistance, T2D, double diabetes, metabolic syndrome, and many associated chronic diseases [Roberts, CK, et al., 2013, Mottalib, A, et al., 2017, Ormazabal, V, et al., 2018]. Acutely, exercise improves insulin sensitivity in both healthy subjects and insulin resistant persons [Heath, GW, et al., 1983]. The improved insulin sensitivity after a single bout of exercise is short-lived (24–72 hours) and declines as each day passes after the exercise bout. Regular exercise training improves insulin sensitivity beyond the acute effect of the last training session. Thus, initiation of a regular exercise program will result in progressively improving insulin sensitivity over 1–2 weeks requiring gradual reductions in insulin doses. With continued regular exercise, insulin doses will stabilize at a new lower dosage. If regular exercise is interrupted or discontinued, insulin doses will need to be gradually increased again.

In order to reap the benefits of exercise while also normalizing blood sugars in those with T1D, we need to first recognize that exercise can be a significant source of variation in blood sugar control if not properly constructed. The blood sugar response to exercise is dependent on three main factors: 1) the current insulin-on-board, meaning how much insulin remains in the subcutaneous fat that has not yet diffused into the bloodstream, 2) the current insulin sensitivity which is dependent on prior bouts of exercise earlier in the day and on previous days, and 3) the degree to which blood sugar-increasing counterregulatory hormones (glucagon, cortisol, epinephrine, and growth hormone) are released during intense exercise. Let's explore these factors affecting the blood sugar response to exercise in more detail.

Insulin-on-Board and the Blood Sugar Response to Exercise

Insulin-on-board includes both basal and bolus insulin whether pumped or injected. Since basal insulin is being released from the subcutaneous injection site continuously, it always represents a potential source of abnormal blood sugars during exercise. By establishing a regular exercise regimen, both basal and BID will automatically be adjusted, as discussed in Chapter 5, to compensate for the effect of the exercise on both insulin sensitivity and counterregulatory hormone release and will result in a reduced need for dextrose supplementation. Basal insulin dosage is adjusted to achieve your target fasting blood sugar. If your fasting blood sugars are low or high, then this can explain low or high blood sugars during and after exercise. The basal insulin dose should be adjusted as discussed in Chapter 5. If your current fasting blood sugars are normal, yet blood sugars during or after exercise are either low or high, then the pre-exercise BID can be decreased or increased, respectively. If you start exercise soon after eating, the exercise diverts blood flow away from the intestines to supply the exercising muscles, increasing the rate of absorption of injected insulin and slowing the rate of nutrient absorption, both of which increase the likelihood of hypoglycemia. You can use the information in Table 5.2 as a guide to judge when to exercise after injecting bolus insulin. Thus, the timing and dosage of basal and mealtime bolus insulin prior to exercise have a significant impact on the occurrence of low or high blood sugars during exercise.

If you can't manage a daily exercise regimen, but can plan exercise prior to bolus insulin injections, the pre-exercise BID can be empirically reduced to avoid hypoglycemia. Post-exercise BID may need to be empirically reduced as well to avoid hypoglycemia. If exercise is completely spontaneous, then pre-exercise, or as needed, dextrose can be consumed to prevent or treat hypoglycemia.

Varying Insulin Sensitivity Adversely Affects Blood Sugars

When insulin sensitivity changes from day to day due to intermittent exercise, we have no way of knowing how much insulin is needed to hit our target blood sugar. I learned this from experience with training for both triathlons and olympic weightlifting. Intermittent exercise, i.e., exercising some days, but not others, leads to more erratic blood sugars compared to steady and consistent exercise day to day. We exercise intermittently either intentionally or spontaneously. For most, it is normal to exercise intermittently when time allows and/or when we feel like doing so. For those who train with an intent to excel at a specific sport, the volume and/or intensity of exercise training often exceeds one's ability to recover by the next day. In this situation, a reduction in training or a rest day is normally suggested to athletes. Training programs called periodization specifically vary exercise volume and intensity to alternate stress and recovery designed to improve athletic performance. In addition to varying volume and intensity on exercise days, rest days and/or 'deload' weeks are prescribed to facilitate recovery. This causes day-to-day variations in insulin sensitivity that makes glycemic control more difficult for those with T1D. Small children normally exercise or play spontaneously and thus incorporating day-to-day consistency is very difficult. As children grow up and can learn the influence of exercise on blood sugars for themselves, a more consistent exercise schedule can gradually be implemented. The improvement in insulin sensitivity due to exercise is beneficial, but it is transient and will wain during the next 24–72 hours. In those who exercise regularly, the improved insulin sensitivity may last up to 10 days after cessation of exercise [Heath, GW, et al., 1983], but will be declining slightly everyday while not exercising. Personally, I have found the improved insulin sensitivity due to exercise begins waning after 24 hours. Usually by dinnertime on the first day of no exercise, I need to start increasing insulin doses to address a high pre-dinner blood sugar from the waning insulin sensitivity. Each subsequent mealtime insulin dose will need to be higher until the next exercise session. Designing a consistent exercise program of daily exercise in the same time-window is the best way to solve this problem. My method to keep insulin sensitivity relatively constant is to perform close to the same exercises, at the same time each day, everyday. Situations that can interfere with accomplishing this are work, school, injury, travel, and other unforeseen life circumstances. To compensate for work/school schedules, a short exercise routine can be done before and/or after work/school, or if possible, during the lunch hour at work. Each session can be short, one aerobic and one resistance, for example. When injury occurs, I adjust to a new set of exercises that does not involve the injured body-part. Inevitably, any change in exercise will affect blood sugar results, but the smaller the change in exercise, the smaller the change in blood sugars. Since we are seeking normal blood sugars rather than perfect blood sugars, changes in exercise beyond our control must be accepted. Similarly when traveling, I design a new exercise routine with the available resources to approximate what I was doing at home. The blood sugar response will not be exactly the same, but will be closer to normal than doing no exercise at all. Some exercise is always better than none in terms of minimizing changes in insulin sensitivity, blood sugars, and insulin doses. In general, increases in physical activity will require immediate reductions in insulin doses and may also require dextrose supplementation to avoid hypoglycemia. Conversely, decreases in physical activity will require increases in insulin doses only after blood sugars begin to increase. If circumstances occur that will not allow for any exercise, your work just won't allow it, or you just don't want to exercise, blood sugars will be easier to manage because insulin sensitivity and counterregulatory hormones will not be varying with exercise.

Intense Exercise Can Release Counterregulatory Hormones

Different types, durations, and intensities of exercise have different effects on blood sugar [Colberg, SR, et al., 2013]. In nondiabetics, blood glucose can temporarily rise above normal after intense exercise due to the release of counterregulatory hormones including epinephrine, glucagon, cortisol, and growth hormone [Thomas, F, et al., 2016]. The body normally releases these hormones in nondiabetics and in those with T1D only during intense exercise to rapidly provide working muscles with fatty acids from the fat cells and glucose and ketones from the liver. It is difficult to know when counterregulatory hormones are the cause of post-exercise high blood sugars without actually measuring them. That said, preventing post-exercise high blood sugars involves designing a consistent exercise plan and adjusting basal and/or pre-exercise insulin doses as previously discussed, or correcting a high blood sugar after exercise with the next scheduled BID.

Consistent Daily Exercise to Achieve Normal Blood Sugars

As mentioned above, intermittent exercise results in daily changes in insulin sensitivity which makes choosing a BID more challenging. Alternatively, eating the same pre-exercise meal and performing the same exercise routine at the same time of day, everyday, facilitates normalizing blood sugars. Designing a consistent daily exercise program was a key strategy that allowed me to finally realize normal blood sugars. This means finding a time slot in your day to do an exercise routine that has the same blood sugar response from day to day. I found that different types of exercise result in different blood sugar responses. For a long time, I was alternating aerobic exercise one day with weightlifting on the next. I assumed my body would appreciate the variation in exercise because it would allow for recovery, but my blood sugars did not. I have experimented with many different combinations of exercise over the years. I found that different aerobic exercises also resulted in different blood sugar responses. For example, swimming was not equivalent to cycling, nor to walking or jogging, in their effect on blood sugar. Similarly, different weightlifting exercises were not equivalent either. Olympic weightlifting did not have the same blood sugar response as weight-machine or bodyweight exercises. For a long time, I resisted repeating the same or very similar exercises everyday due to concerns about overtraining and/or an inability to recover, but my desire to normalize my blood sugars inspired me to try it anyway. It turned out to be quite successful in every respect and I can make small improvements from day to day while maintaining normal blood sugars in the process.

Circumstances can arise that cause an interruption in one's exercise routine. When the interruption is expected to be less than one week, I have found just increasing the BID in response to increasing blood sugars results in close to normal glycemic control compared to increasing both basal and BID. When the interruption in exercise is expected to be more than one week, I have found that insulin sensitivity wanes enough that an increase in the basal insulin dose, due to an increase in fasting blood glucose, is needed, in addition to increasing the bolus doses, to restore normal blood sugars.

If consistent daily exercise is just not an option for you, or in the case of small children, taking pre-exercise dextrose, as needed, is another method to prevent exercise-related hypoglycemia. Keeping track of how much dextrose is used allows one to make adjustments to result in normal or near-normal blood glucose during and after exercise. I suggest carrying dextrose with you at all times including during exercise. I have regretted not having dextrose readily available in the past. I do not hesitate consuming dextrose anytime I don't feel quite right. When I was training for triathlons, I carried my blood glucose meter to check my blood sugar every hour. I can appreciate that having a CGM when exercising for long periods of time would have been more convenient. Keep in mind that CGM can be less accurate during exercise as discussed in Chapter 6.

How to Structure Your Exercise Plan

The first step in developing your own exercise plan is to find a time each day when you can exercise. Then choose an exercise you like, otherwise, you are not likely to continue with it. All types of exercise are beneficial, but if you can manage to do some aerobic and resistance exercise, that is best for overall health. You can do both resistance and aerobic exercise back to back or schedule them in different time slots in your day. This study [Yardley, JE, et al., 2012] concluded that "Performing resistance exercise before aerobic exercise improved glycemic stability throughout exercise and reduced the duration and severity of post-exercise hypoglycemia for individuals with T1D." By sticking with a consistent exercise regimen, basal and bolus insulin does can be adjusted to compensate for the activity. This is the key to avoiding low and high blood sugars while minimizing the need to take dextrose. If you can only do 15 mins of activity, that is fine. Something is always better than nothing. Once you adapt to 15 mins, you can increase it at your own pace if you desire. Increasing duration, volume, or intensity of exercise gradually over time is recommended to improve fitness and strength over time [2018 Physical Activity Guidelines Advisory Committee, 2nd edition, 2018]. Having a gym membership or gym equipment is not required to participate in both aerobic and resistance exercise. Walking, pushups, air squats, lunges, or climbing stairs are examples of aerobic and resistance exercises that can be done for free without exercise equipment. By searching YouTube for 'bodyweight exercises no equipment' you can find numerous exercises demonstrated for you. Yoga is a combination of resistance, balance, and flexibility training with a meditation component.

Yoga can be done at home and you can find YouTube videos of workouts to follow or you can join a local class that adds social interaction as well. Strength and balance training is recommended for older adults to help prevent falls. Falls in older adults are common, ≈ 29% of adults over age 65 fall each year and lead to major injuries, e.g., bone fractures and head trauma, early death, and considerable medical expense [Bergen, G, et al., 2016]. The frequency of falls in older adults was reduced with a home-based strength and balance exercise program [Liu-Ambrose, T, et al., 2019].

If you have flexibility in the time slot(s) during which you exercise, I would suggest waiting 2–3 hours after a meal so that most of the meal nutrients and mealtime bolus insulin has already been absorbed into the bloodstream. This will decrease the likelihood of hypoglycemia. Many busy people get up early in the morning to exercise before breakfast, but in some, this can result in abnormal blood sugars. Low blood sugars can be prevented or corrected with dextrose and high blood sugars can be corrected with a small dose of bolus insulin. If breakfast follows the early morning exercise, the BID can be adjusted to take the exercise into account. Measuring blood glucose with a meter or CGM is a good idea during long endurance training sessions to detect impending hypoglycemia and to understand your blood glucose response to any dextrose taken.

In summary, exercise is very beneficial and I would say essential if you want to maximize your health-span. When performed on an irregular basis, exercise does make managing blood sugars more difficult for those with T1D. However, simply planning a regular daily exercise program along with consistent LCD meals allows for BID to be more predictable and result in normal blood sugars.

Compensating for Exercise in Children

Keeping exercise consistent from day to day is difficult for young children to comply with. If possible, the parent/caregiver can estimate, relative to the previous day, the amount/intensity of physical activity and observe the post-exercise blood glucose results to base subsequent BID relative to those given on the previous days. Pre-exercise dextrose is a good option to prevent hypoglycemia during exercise and sometimes post-exercise dextrose is necessary as well. If possible, the child, or the parent/caregiver depending on the child's age, can record the type and amount of physical activity, the quantity of dextrose consumed, and the resulting pre- and post-exercise blood glucose, for future dextrose-dosing decisions. As mentioned above, different activities will have different effects on blood glucose and will require different amounts of dextrose to maintain normal blood sugars. Post-exercise insulin doses may need to be reduced to prevent hypoglycemia which can occur at night while sleeping. This is a situation where a CGM with alarm capability can be a life-saving tool in children.

Avoiding Exercise-Related Hypoglycemia

The fear of exercise-related hypoglycemia a significant factor in deterring those with T1D from participating in exercise [Colberg, SR, et al., 2015]. I was afraid of exercise-related hypoglycemia while training for triathlons and consequently took more sugar, and later dextrose, than I actually needed resulting in high blood sugars. Nevertheless, I would not let my initial errors stop me from pursuing exercise. Instead, I experimented with bolus and basal insulin dose reductions, more frequent blood glucose measurements, and more prudent dextrose supplementation to prevent exercise-related hypoglycemia. After beginning my VLCD, I experienced a marked reduction in exercise-related hypoglycemia which allowed me to further reduce my dextrose supplementation before and during exercise. This was likely due to a combination of 1) reduced insulin doses, 2) increased muscular fat utilization [Volek, JS, et al., 2016], and 3) reduced muscular glucose utilization, due to the glucose/fatty acid cycle, described in 1963 [Dimitriadis, G, et al., 2011]. Hypoglycemia after exercise can result from continued glucose uptake by muscles or an excessive post-exercise BID. This is especially dangerous when it occurs while sleeping when one's awareness of hypoglycemia is impaired. This is where a CGM can be a valuable tool in alerting those with T1D and their partners/parents/caregivers of impending nocturnal hypoglycemia.

In summary, aerobic, resistance, and HIIT exercise can and should be enjoyed by those with T1D without the fear of hypoglycemia. Consistency of exercise day to day is the most powerful strategy to avoid hypoglycemia with minimal dextrose consumption while still achieving normal blood sugars. Reducing pre-exercise BID, properly adjusting basal insulin doses, consuming dextrose prior to and during exercise, as needed, and using a CGM with alarm capability to detect impending hypoglycemia are effective strategies to prevent exercise-associated hypoglycemia.

8 – Sleep, Sunshine, Alcohol & Tobacco

"There is a time for many words, and there is also a time for sleep."
Homer, The Odyssey.

"He who is not courageous enough to take risks will accomplish nothing in life."
Muhammad Ali, "The Greatest," professional boxer.

Sleep, Sunshine, and Circadian Rhythms

Sleep is a restorative process for our body and brain that is essential for optimal health. Insufficient sleep duration and poor sleep quality result in numerous adverse effects including disturbed metabolic health, worsening insulin sensitivity, increased insulin requirements, and cravings for unhealthful foods. Glucose metabolism and insulin sensitivity also vary throughout the day due to our circadian rhythm [Reinke, H, et al., 2019]. In those with T1D, mealtime insulin doses will vary throughout the day, in part, due to our circadian rhythm. Shift-work, jet lag, and other circadian-clock disruptions can increase ghrelin, hunger, and food cravings and are associated with detrimental effects on nutrient metabolism resulting in higher post-meal blood glucose, insulin resistance, hyperinsulinemia, metabolic syndrome, obesity, T2D, and likely double diabetes in those with T1D.

This study measured blood glucose, insulin, glucagon, liver glucose production, muscle glucose uptake, and liver insulin extraction throughout the day in 20 metabolically healthy subjects in response to breakfast, lunch, and dinner meals of identical macronutrients in a research laboratory [Saad, A, et al., 2012]. The purpose was to understand if a diurnal pattern to insulin secretion and responsiveness existed across the day to help design artificial pancreas device control algorithms for those with T1D. The study was carefully done to eliminate variations in the timing of meals, meal macronutrients, and timing and amount of physical activity. The increase in post-meal blood glucose was significantly lower at breakfast than lunch and dinner. Pancreatic β-cell insulin secretion was more rapid and to a greater extent at breakfast than lunch and dinner. The subjects were more insulin sensitive at breakfast compared to lunch or dinner. This study suggests the existence of a diurnal pattern to insulin secretion, responsiveness to insulin, and the post-meal blood sugar response in healthy humans. I would like to point out that the authors of this study recognized the importance of eliminating as many variables as possible to be able to accurately assess the subject's response to insulin. These variables included the timing of meals, quantity of meal macronutrients, and timing and amount of physical activity. This coincides precisely with my method of treating T1D since normalizing blood sugars requires a precise match between exogenous insulin dosages, meal macronutrients, and insulin sensitivity related to exercise.

Our circadian rhythm is regulated by both adequate daytime sunlight exposure and the absence of blue-light exposure after sundown. Since learning of the impact of sleep on insulin sensitivity, I adjusted my sleep schedule to go to bed at 10:30 PM and wake up at 7 AM each day. I also keep my room dark and cool without electronic devices to disturb me. After sundown, I utilize a blue-light wavelength blocking app (f.lux) on my computer and shut it off completely 2–3 hours before bedtime. This aids in getting a good night's sleep because post-sundown blue-light inhibits melatonin secretion. Melatonin is a hormone secreted by the pineal gland in the brain which serves to initiate and maintain sleep. Night-time levels of melatonin are normally at least 10-times higher than daytime concentrations with proper sleep hygiene habits [Rzepka-Migut, B, et al., 2020]. Getting prudent sunlight exposure, i.e., not burning, during the day properly regulates our circadian clock as well as producing vitamin D3 in the skin especially when that exposure occurs around the noon hour when UVB rays are at a maximum. UVB rays also stimulate production of melanin, the brown pigment in skin cells, that causes tanning (increased pigmentation) and also protects our skin cell's DNA from ultraviolet radiation damage. UVA rays, present throughout the daylight hours, promote nitric oxide production in the skin which lowers blood pressure. Thus, there are multiple benefits of regular, but prudent, sun exposure.

Sleep hygiene habits that facilitate restorative sleep include:
1. Keep a regular schedule of bedtime and wake-time.
2. Use blue-light blocking apps on electronic devices after sunset.
3. Keep bedroom dark, cool, and gadget-free.
4. Avoid caffeine 6–8 hours before bedtime.
5. Exercise daily, but complete it 2–3 hours before bedtime.
6. Nicotine, alcohol, and numerous over-the-counter and prescription medications can interfere with sleep, talk with your physician about your medications.
7. Get a prudent amount of daily natural sunlight exposure.

Alcohol Use In Those With Diabetes

This review article [Emanuele, NV, et al., 1998] explains the effects of alcohol on those with and without diabetes. I have selected pertinent quotes from this review article that explain why I believe those with diabetes should consider abstaining from alcohol if optimal health is their primary goal.

"Because alcohol use, at least on a social level, is widespread among diabetics as well as nondiabetics, clinicians and researchers must understand alcohol's effect on the progression and complications of diabetes. First, alcohol consumption can lead to a situation called hypoglycemic unawareness in both diabetics and nondiabetics. Second, diabetics who have consumed alcohol, particularly those with T1D, experience a delayed glucose recovery from hypoglycemia. The combination of alcohol-induced hypoglycemia, hypoglycemic unawareness, and delayed recovery from hypoglycemia can lead to deleterious health consequences. Heavy alcohol consumption (i.e., 200 grams of pure alcohol, or approximately 16 standard drinks, per day) can cause ketoacidosis in both diabetics and nondiabetics. Diabetes and alcohol consumption are the two most common underlying causes of peripheral neuropathy. All of these findings suggest that alcohol and diabetes can enhance each other's effects in terms of causing nerve damage. In people with diabetes, the pancreas does not produce sufficient insulin, T1D, or the body does not respond appropriately to the insulin, T2D. Alcohol consumption by diabetics can worsen blood sugar control in those patients. For example, long-term alcohol use in well-nourished diabetics can result in excessive blood sugar levels. Conversely, long-term alcohol ingestion in diabetics who are not adequately nourished can lead to dangerously low blood sugar levels. Finally, alcohol consumption can worsen diabetes-related medical complications, such as disturbances in fat metabolism, nerve damage, and eye disease. Regular consumption of even moderate amounts of alcohol (i.e., two to four drinks per day), however, clearly interferes with diabetic blood sugar control and increases the risk of impotence; peripheral neuropathy; and, possibly, retinopathy."

Tobacco Use In Those With Diabetes

In 2018, 13.7% of Americans were smoking tobacco. For those with T1D, smoking is particularly dangerous and I would encourage you to quit smoking if you do. Smoking worsens all of the long-term diabetic complications: retinopathy (eye disease), nephropathy (kidney disease), neuropathy (nerve disease), and CVD. This study [Chaturvedi, N, et al., 1995] concluded that, "Smoking is associated with poorer glycemic control and an increased prevalence of microvascular complications compared with not smoking. Ex-smokers can achieve glycemic control equivalent to and have a prevalence of early complications similar to that of those who never smoked. We suggest that poorer glycemic control can account for some of the increased risk of complications in smokers, and that quitting smoking would be effective in reducing the incidence of complications. Urgent action is required to reduce the high smoking rates in people with IDDM (insulin dependent diabetes mellitus)."

In a similar study [Braffett, BH, et al., 2019b] of patients in the Diabetes Control and Complications Trial (DCCT 1983–1993), the authors concluded that, "During a mean of 6.5 years of follow-up, current smokers had consistently higher HbA1c values and were at a higher risk of retinopathy and nephropathy compared with former and never smokers. These risk differences were attenuated after adjusting for HbA1c suggesting that the negative association of smoking on glycemic control is partially responsible for the adverse association of smoking on the risk of complications in T1D. Current smokers had a 43% increased risk of retinopathy compared with never smokers and a 36% increased risk of nephropathy. These findings support the potential for a beneficial effect of smoking cessation on complications in T1D."

9 – Medications & Hormones Affecting Blood Sugars

"Knowledge is power"
Francis Bacon, English philosopher and statesman.

"The greater the ignorance, the greater the dogmatism."
Sir William Osler, MDCM, a founding father of modern medicine,
Johns Hopkins University.

Medications

The following are examples of medications that may accentuate the blood-glucose-lowering effect of insulin and, therefore, increase one's susceptibility to hypoglycemia: oral diabetes medications, pramlintide acetate, angiotensin converting enzyme (ACE) inhibitors, disopyramide, fibrates, fluoxetine, monoamine oxidase (MAO) inhibitors, propoxyphene, pentoxifylline, salicylates, somatostatin analogs, and sulfonamide antibiotics.

On the contrary, the following medications can reduce the blood-glucose-lowering effect of insulin: corticosteroids (synthetic forms of cortisol), niacin, danazol, diuretics, sympathomimetic agents (e.g., epinephrine, albuterol, terbutaline), glucagon, isoniazid, phenothiazine derivatives, somatropin, thyroid hormones, oral contraceptives (e.g., estrogen/progesterone), protease inhibitors, and atypical antipsychotic medications (e.g., olanzapine and clozapine).

Other classes of medications that can alter glucose metabolism include antibiotics, antipsychotics, beta-blockers, calcineurin and protease inhibitors, and thiazide diuretics. Beta-blockers, clonidine, lithium salts, and alcohol may either increase or decrease the blood-glucose-lowering effect of insulin. Pentamidine can cause hypoglycemia, which may sometimes be followed by hyperglycemia. The signs and symptoms of hypoglycemia can be reduced or absent in patients taking blood-pressure-lowering anti-adrenergic drugs such as beta-blockers, clonidine, guanethidine, and reserpine.

Large doses of vitamin C given intravenously can interfere with the measurement of blood glucose in home blood glucose meters that use glucose oxidase-based strips, e.g., OneTouch, without actually changing blood glucose levels. If you receive a large dose of vitamin C and find that soon afterwards your blood glucose is quite elevated, you should use a home blood glucose meter that uses glucose dehydrogenase-flavin adenine dinucleotide-based strips, e.g., Bayer Contour Next [Vasudevan, S, et al., 2014]. If you are not aware of or ignore this and treat a falsely-elevated blood glucose reading with additional insulin, you may induce hypoglycemia.

The above does not mean you should never take any of these medications, only that you should be aware of their potential to affect your blood glucose readings or the signs and symptoms of hypoglycemia. You should review all of your medications with your physician to improve your understanding of their potential to adversely affect your blood sugar control.

SGLT2 Inhibitors

SGLT2 inhibitors (Sodium-glucose cotransporter-2) are a newer class of medications approved by the FDA in the U.S. for the treatment of T2D. They are occasionally prescribed 'off-label' to those with poorly-controlled T1D. Drugs in this class of medications include canagliflozin (Invokana), dapagliflozin (Farxiga), empagliflozin (Jardiance), and ipragliflozin (currently only in Japan). SGLT2 inhibitors work by blocking the kidney's ability to reabsorb filtered glucose, allowing the glucose to escape into the urine (glycosuria). This mechanism of action is dependent on the current blood glucose level and is independent of the action of insulin [Kalra, S, 2014].

When used for T1D, SGLT2 inhibitors potently lower blood glucose requiring a reduction in daily insulin dose. While a reduction in insulin dose is beneficial, SGLT2 inhibitors also increase glucagon secretion by the α-cells which, in turn, stimulates liver glucose and ketone production. There have been several reports of DKA or euglycemic DKA (euDKA), meaning DKA with a blood glucose < 200 mg/dl (11.1 mM), in patients with T1D taking SGLT2 inhibitors [Peters, AL, et al., 2015, Rosenstock, J, et al., 2015, Wolfsdorf, JI, et al., 2019]. In euDKA caused by SGLT2 inhibitors, liver ketone production is accelerated while elevation in blood glucose is prevented by the loss of glucose in the urine. Because blood glucose is not particularly elevated in euDKA, those with T1D would not normally suspect that they were developing DKA, and therefore, may delay seeking medical attention. In a phase 3 clinical trial [Danne, T, et al., 2019] of a new SGLT1+2 inhibitor, sotagliflozin, the authors state: "As a general guideline, SGLT inhibitor therapy should not be used in patients using low-carbohydrate or ketogenic diets as, anecdotally, they seem to be at increased risk of adverse ketosis effects and certainly create a diagnostic dilemma in evaluating the clinical significance of ketosis. Also, with regard to diet, patients who skip meals and/or consume excessive alcohol seem to be at increased risk [of DKA]."

Stress Hormones

Stress hormones including cortisol, epinephrine, growth hormone, and glucagon signal fat cells to release fatty acids and the liver to release glucose and ketones. These catabolic counterregulatory hormones can be appropriately elevated by stressful situations like intense exercise, illness (e.g., infection), trauma, surgery, and intense heat or cold. This is obviously beneficial in the short-term, but for those with T1D, the increase in blood glucose will need to be corrected with exogenous insulin. Chronic stress, often encountered in modern life, is not beneficial and can cause insulin resistance and increases in blood sugar. Chronic stress should be addressed with any modality that helps to manage it including exercise, meditation, massage, counseling, social connections, changing your job, location, partner, friends, and/or living situation. The increase in stress hormones related to exercise is limited in extent and duration and one post-exercise correction insulin bolus, typically with the post-exercise meal, is enough to correct the post-exercise hyperglycemia. By contrast, the stress hormone increase due to illness is often to a greater extent and duration. Caution should be exercised to prevent excessive increases in bolus and basal dosages to achieve normal blood sugars in a hurry. It is safer to accept mildly elevated blood sugars, e.g., 130–180 mg/dl (7.2–10.0 mM), during an illness to prevent life-threatening hypoglycemia while monitoring blood ketone levels. BID should be carefully increased when blood sugars exceed 180 mg/dl (10.0 mM) to prevent DKA. This is another situation where you should involve your physician in your blood sugar management.

Hormonal Changes During Menstrual Cycles

In nondiabetic premenopausal women, pancreatic β-cell insulin release as well as estrogen and progesterone secretion vary throughout the menstrual cycle resulting in varying insulin sensitivity without significant change in blood sugar. The length of a menstrual cycle is the number of days between the first day of menstrual bleeding (menses) of one cycle to the onset of menses of the next cycle. The median duration of a menstrual cycle is 28 days with most cycle lengths between 25 to 30 days. The menstrual cycle can be divided into two phases: 1) the follicular or proliferative phase, and 2) the luteal or secretory phase. The follicular phase begins from the first day of menses until ovulation. The development of ovarian follicles characterizes this phase, one of which will mature and release an egg which travels down the fallopian tube to the uterus. A surge in luteinizing hormone (LH) is initiated by a dramatic rise of estradiol produced by the preovulatory follicle and results in subsequent ovulation. The LH surge also stimulates the synthesis of progesterone responsible for the midcycle follicle stimulating hormone (FSH) surge. The luteal phase is 14 days long in most women. If the egg is not fertilized, progesterone levels decline and results in menses. The average duration of menstrual bleeding is 4–6 days [Reed, BG, et al., 2018]. This study [Yeung, EH, et al., 2010] of 257 healthy premenopausal women found that HOMA-IR, a measure of insulin resistance, increased from 1.35 during the midfollicular phase to 1.59 during the early luteal phase, an 18% increase, and decreased to 1.55 in the late-luteal phase. Some menstruating women with T1D will experience monthly cyclical changes characterized by increasing blood sugars after the start of ovulation and decreasing blood sugars after the start of menstruation. The timing of these changes in blood sugars are not usually able to be precisely anticipated so insulin doses must be increased, and then decreased, in response to the actual blood glucose readings. In addition, the estrogen in birth control pills can raise blood glucose levels and increase insulin resistance requiring an increase in exogenous insulin doses [Cortés, ME, et al., 2014]. In this case, the pattern of blood sugar changes may be more predictable since the birth control pills are taken on a regular schedule.

10 – Hypoglycemia

"When the going gets tough, the tough get going."
John Thomas, Texas football coach.

"Insulin is a remedy that is primarily for the wise and not the foolish, be they patients or doctors."
Elliott P. Joslin, MD, America's first diabetologist.

"The best things in life, aren't things."
Various attributions.

Hypoglycemia in Type 1 Diabetes

Having had T1D since 1998, I can definitely say that hypoglycemia is the most undesirable and dangerous aspect of having T1D. Hypoglycemia frequently occupies the mind of those with T1D. When it occurs, we feel anywhere from unpleasant to panic-stricken. When in the company of others, it is embarrassing due to one's inability to prevent it and becoming the center of attention, especially if one's behavior changes. When recurrent, it imposes not only on our lives, but also on the lives of family members. When severe, it can cause injury during seizures, permanent disability from brain damage, or death. Hypoglycemia often causes ill-defined post-hypoglycemic symptoms that last for hours possibly related to counterregulatory hormone release and the hyperglycemia that results. Over the years, my distain of hypoglycemia has inspired me to develop a more thorough understanding of the causes, symptoms, dangers, treatment, and most importantly, the prevention of hypoglycemia.

Hypoglycemia occurs when too much exogenous insulin is administered relative to one's current needs. This occurs primarily because of the difficulty in predicting the exact insulin dose that is needed at any given time. Once hypoglycemia does occur in those with T1D, the physiological response, meaning the liver's ability to raise blood glucose, is impaired, and the behavioral response, meaning our ability to recognize and treat hypoglycemia with dextrose, is impaired in those with hypoglycemia unawareness. As you have learned so far, a LCD/VLCD with day-to-day consistency and timing of meals, meal macronutrients, exercise, and sleep are key elements that make dosing insulin more predictable. If you can utilize these strategies, I believe hypoglycemia will be an unusual occurrence for you as it is for me now. I am highly motivated to continue my current lifestyle simply to avoid hypoglycemia and enjoy normal blood sugars. It is difficult to communicate to those without T1D the utter relief that comes from not having to worry about impending hypoglycemia, or to deal with its consequences, or to accept the long-term diabetic complications that result from maintaining high blood sugars simply to avoid hypoglycemia.

The average T1D patient suffers one episode of severe hypoglycemia, often with seizure or coma per year, two episodes of symptomatic hypoglycemia per week, and an untold number of asymptomatic hypoglycemic episodes. When using conventional nutritional guidelines (LFHCD) combined with intensive insulin therapy, hypoglycemia becomes the limiting factor in the glycemic management of T1D. Hypoglycemia precludes the maintenance of normal blood sugars and thus the ability to prevent complications of diabetes over a lifetime. Hypoglycemia is the primary reason professional diabetes associations do not recommend normal blood sugars, although if it could be accomplished safely, would undoubtedly be beneficial with respect to the long-term complications of diabetes [Cryer, PE, 2012].

The brain adapts to hypoglycemia with as few as one episode of hypoglycemia by lowering the blood glucose threshold needed to evoke the symptoms of hypoglycemia. The medical term for this phenomenon is 'hypoglycemia unawareness,' although a more precise term is 'impaired awareness of hypoglycemia.' Hypoglycemia unawareness occurs in ≈ 40% of those with T1D and results in a six-fold greater risk of severe hypoglycemia [Martín-Timón, I, et al., 2015]. In this condition, hypoglycemia begets more hypoglycemia, creating a viscous cycle. This translates to increasingly frequent asymptomatic and symptomatic hypoglycemic episodes and their potential for harm. Because the blood sugar at which symptoms of hypoglycemia appear depends on the presence or absence of hypoglycemia unawareness, I will define hypoglycemia as any blood glucose < 70 mg/dl (3.9 mM). That said, symptoms of hypoglycemia can occur at blood glucose levels > 70 mg/dl (3.9 mM) when the brain has adapted to chronically elevated blood sugars as in those with poorly-controlled T1D. For these individuals, their target blood sugar should be set high enough to avoid symptomatic hypoglycemia. Over time, with improved glycemic control, one's target blood glucose can be reduced. The brain will adapt to normal blood glucose levels and symptoms will only occur when the blood glucose is < 70 mg/dl (3.9 mM).

My highest priority in treating T1D is to avoid hypoglycemia even if that means other goals are not quite met. Because hypoglycemia is so dangerous, I suggest everyone with T1D make its avoidance their highest priority as well.

Physiologic Response to Hypoglycemia

In nondiabetic individuals, as blood glucose falls to 80–85 mg/dl (4.4–4.7 mM), the β-cells stop secreting insulin. Once blood glucose falls to 65–70 mg/dl (3.6–3.9 mM), the α-cells increase glucagon secretion, the autonomic sympathetic nerves begin secreting norepinephrine and acetylcholine, the adrenal glands begin secreting epinephrine, norepinephrine, and cortisol, and the pituitary gland secretes growth hormone. Glucagon stimulates liver glucose production which increases blood glucose. Epinephrine stimulates glucose production in both the liver and kidneys to a greater extent than that of glucagon. Cortisol and growth hormone increase liver glucose production, but their effects are delayed and prolonged.

In persons with T1D, the normal reduction in β-cell insulin secretion does not occur and exogenous insulin levels remain elevated during hypoglycemia. The α-cells, in turn, are not signaled to secrete glucagon due to the high exogenous insulin levels. Thus, these two physiologic mechanisms that normally raise blood glucose levels are absent in those with T1D. Epinephrine and norepinephrine signal the liver and kidneys to produce glucose and, along with acetylcholine, cause the symptoms of hypoglycemia that implore those with T1D to ingest carbohydrate (dextrose), which together, increases blood glucose. Counterregulatory hormone and neurotransmitter secretion can lead to post-hypoglycemic hyperglycemia as can the excessive treatment of hypoglycemia with carbohydrate.

Symptomatic Response to Hypoglycemia

In the absence of hypoglycemia unawareness, symptoms of hypoglycemia typically appear as the blood glucose falls to 50–55 mg/dl (2.8–3.1 mM). Brain function becomes impaired with reduced cognitive ability, aberrant behavior, seizure, and coma as the blood glucose falls below 50 mg/dl (2.8 mM). Brain death occurs when the blood glucose falls below 20 mg/dl (1.1 mM) due to functional brain failure [Cryer, PE, 2012]. Hypoglycemic neurogenic symptoms caused by the secretion of epinephrine and norepinephrine include palpitations, increased heart rate, tremor, anxiety, and increased arousal. The secretion of acetylcholine causes sweating, hunger, and paresthesias (numbness of skin). Neuroglycopenic symptoms occur as a direct result of brain glucose deprivation and include cognitive impairments (memory, attention, and information processing) [Graveling, AJ, et al., 2013], behavioral changes, and psychomotor abnormalities (uncontrolled body movements).

Any feeling you have that is out of the ordinary or occurs in a different context, e.g., feeling sleepy at a time when you normally do not, could be a symptom of hypoglycemia. It is prudent to check your blood sugar or if you don't have that capability at the moment, then take dextrose to ensure your safety. Signs and symptoms of hypoglycemia that have been reported by those with T1D, many of which I have experienced myself, include anxiety, nervousness, appearing pale, awakening from sleep, blurred vision, coma, confusion, denial of hypoglycemia, dizziness, double vision, dropping objects, fatigue, weakness, headache, hunger, inability to sleep, inappropriate laughter, irritability, lightheadedness, and nasty behavior. Additional symptoms include nausea, nightmares, numbness of skin, panic, fear of death, pounding heartbeat, profuse sweating, rapid heartbeat, ringing in ears, seeing spots or lights, seizure, sleepiness, stubbornness, uncontrolled movements, and visual hallucinations.

The Dangers of Hypoglycemia & Hypoglycemia Unawareness

Hypoglycemia is very dangerous for those with T1D as evidenced by the fact that anywhere from 4% to 10% will die from hypoglycemia [Skrivarhaug, T, et al., 2006]. Hypoglycemia unawareness results from 1) one or more recent hypoglycemic episodes, 2) drinking alcohol, 3) exercise, and 4) sleep. Therefore, one should avoid having hypoglycemic episodes, alcohol, and use extra caution when choosing post-exercise and pre-sleep insulin doses during these more vulnerable times. In those with hypoglycemia unawareness, the neurologic adaptation to hypoglycemia results in reduced release of epinephrine [Reno, CM, et al., 2013] causing fewer or no neurogenic symptoms to occur as the blood glucose falls to 50–55 mg/dl (2.8–3.1 mM). When the blood glucose falls below 50 mg/dl (2.8 mM), neuroglycopenia can cause those with T1D to be less aware of neurogenic symptoms, delaying or preventing one from taking dextrose, which makes hypoglycemia unawareness a dangerous condition. This explains why some with T1D are found dead-in-bed [Secrest, AM, et al., 2011]. They were likely not awoken by hypoglycemia due to the absence or paucity of neurogenic symptoms, quickly transitioned to neuroglycopenia, and were unable to recognize the few hypoglycemic symptoms they may have had while sleeping. In other words, they went to sleep and were never aware they were hypoglycemic. Detection of nocturnal hypoglycemia is the most valuable attribute of using a CGM with alarm capability especially if another individual in the house can be alerted simultaneously.

Personal examples of neuroglycopenia that I experienced during a hypoglycemic episode that delayed its treatment include: 1) not noticing I was sweating, 2) thinking my sweating was appropriate, 3) not remembering a drive home from work, and 4) being argumentative with my wife when she told me I was hypoglycemic and needed to take dextrose. Once I told her she should take dextrose! Even remembering what I did during these hypoglycemic episodes is embarrassing. Thus, you should not take any comfort in not having symptoms of hypoglycemia when the blood glucose falls below 55 mg/dl (3.1 mM). Instead, this should be your warning that you are experiencing hypoglycemia unawareness and you need to make adjustments in your treatment of T1D to avoid hypoglycemia altogether. You should determine whether basal, bolus, or both insulin preparations should be reduced, the times they should be reduced, and by how much the dose(s) should be reduced. Fortunately, hypoglycemia unawareness is a reversible condition by avoiding all hypoglycemia for a period of 2–3 weeks and is preventable by avoiding further hypoglycemia [Fanelli, CG, et al., 1993].

On December 18, 2015, I wrote blog post #12 at https://ketogenicdiabeticathlete.wordpress.com/2015/12/18/hypoglycemia-can-ketones-help-fuel-the-brain/, to explore the idea that nutritional ketosis might produce enough ketones to explain the development of asymptomatic hypoglycemia which I first noticed within one week after starting my VLCD in 2012 without any change in blood glucose readings. However, this study published after I wrote that blog post [see Fig. 7D in Cunnane, SC, et al., 2016] indicates that a blood ketone concentration of 1.5 mM, typical of nutritional ketosis, can only supply enough energy for ≈ 20% of brain metabolism. Thus, hypoglycemia unawareness, rather than brain utilization of ketones, is the explanation for asymptomatic hypoglycemia in those with T1D in nutritional ketosis by following a

VLCD. The proper response to asymptomatic hypoglycemia is to avoid hypoglycemia altogether. There are no known benefits of hypoglycemia, but numerous known harms. For many years, I did not think it was even possible to make hypoglycemia a rare event, but now I do. By following the strategies in this book and carefully and conservatively dosing insulin, we can minimize or avoid blood glucose readings < 70 mg/dl (< 3.9 mM) which will ensure our safety. Avoiding hypoglycemia should be our highest priority in the treatment of T1D.

Treatment of Hypoglycemia

The most effective way to treat hypoglycemia is with pure glucose, also called dextrose. Dextrose comes in either tablet (4 grams/tablet) or liquid form. In the U.S. and Canada, a candy called Smarties™ is an inexpensive form of dextrose (6 grams/roll). I think many with T1D, myself included, have made the mistake of trying to take advantage of a hypoglycemic episode by eating a sweet treat that they know they can't normally eat. This is not an effective way to treat hypoglycemia because sweet foods or sweet treats usually contain sucrose and fat which will not raise blood glucose nearly as fast as pure dextrose. This delays the resolution of your symptoms causing you to eat more than is needed to raise your blood glucose to a normal level and often results in hyperglycemia. Because sugars are not absorbed in the mouth, esophagus, or stomach, there is a time delay before the dextrose reaches the small intestine where it is absorbed. When dextrose is taken to treat hypoglycemia, it takes ≈ 15 mins to be absorbed and as much as ≈ 30 mins before the symptoms of hypoglycemia are noticeably improved. I have found drinking some water seems to help move the dextrose to the small intestine a bit quicker. This time delay makes it difficult to resist overdosing on dextrose, let alone, a sweet treat. The ADA recommends the 15-15 rule to treat hypoglycemia.

Consume 15 grams of rapid-acting carbohydrate (four dextrose tablets) and check a finger-stick blood glucose after 15 mins. If it's still below 70 mg/dl (3.9 mM), have another serving. Repeat these steps until your blood glucose is at least 70 mg/dl (3.9 mM). Each person will need to experiment with the quantity and timing of dextrose ingestion to correct hypoglycemia without causing hyperglycemia. One hypoglycemic symptom, panic or fear-of-death, can compel one to over-consume dextrose. I don't have a solution for that problem except to avoid hypoglycemia in the first place. The number of dextrose tablets I have used over the years varies quite a bit from as few as two (8 grams of dextrose) to as many as six (24 grams dextrose) without causing hyperglycemia. The ADA recommends eating some protein-food after correcting hypoglycemia to reduce the likelihood of another episode due to the continued absorption of previously injected insulin.

It is prudent to always carry dextrose with you at all times. Obviously, if you find yourself with hypoglycemic symptoms and have not brought your dextrose with you, get the next best available option whether it is table sugar, sucrose, or food. Foods that can raise blood glucose more quickly than others include grapes, raisins, fruit juice, and non-diet sodas. Remember the dose matters. You want enough to raise your blood sugar, but you also want to avoid overdoing it and ending-up with a sky-high blood glucose afterwards. Checking your blood glucose before and after treatment of hypoglycemia can help you judge how much dextrose you will need in the future. If you don't have your meter with you, it is perfectly acceptable to treat suspected hypoglycemia with dextrose.

Baqsimi is the first glucagon therapy approved for the emergency treatment of severe hypoglycemia that can be administered without an injection. Baqsimi is a powder administered into the nose of a person experiencing severe hypoglycemia who is unable to eat and swallow dextrose. Baqsimi increases blood glucose levels by stimulating the liver to release stored glucose into the bloodstream. You will need to ask your physician for a prescription.

I am occasionally asked, 'Does treating hypoglycemia with dextrose knock you out of nutritional ketosis?' The answer is: 'I haven't measured my ketones after treating hypoglycemia, so I don't know. For the sake of discussion, if it did, the excess exogenous insulin that caused the hypoglycemia would be responsible for doing so, not the dextrose. The mechanism whereby dextrose (or any carbohydrate) inhibits ketone synthesis is via stimulation of β-cell insulin secretion, which of course, does not happen in those with T1D. Insulin inhibits ketone production by several mechanisms including inhibiting the rate-limiting enzyme, HMG-CoA synthase, in ketone synthesis. Thus, if nutritional ketosis were abolished, it would be due to the excess exogenous insulin that caused the hypoglycemia, not the dextrose used to treat it.' I fear the reasoning behind this question is that some may feel treating hypoglycemia with dextrose might reduce ketones which could be used by the brain in place of dextrose. This is flawed logic since, as mentioned above, nutritional ketosis can't provide the brain with enough ketones to support brain function in the setting of hypoglycemia.

Prevention of Hypoglycemia

Preventing hypoglycemia should be our highest priority in the treatment of T1D. Reducing the frequency of hypoglycemia is an inherent result of implementing the strategies in this book. A LCD/VLCD combined with meal, exercise, and sleep consistency all contribute to reducing hypoglycemia and the variability of blood sugars via more predictable insulin dosing. When hypoglycemia does occur, it is very important to take the time to analyze why it may have occurred and make appropriate adjustments to your lifestyle regimen and/or insulin-dosing decisions to prevent it. You should also consult with your physician to help understand the cause(s) of hypoglycemia if it is not readily apparent to you. There is always a reason for hypoglycemia, and while it may not always be preventable, it is not an inevitable part of treating T1D with exogenous insulin.

Possible reasons for hypoglycemia include:
1. A recent reduction in food intake.
2. A recent reduction in bodyweight.
3. A recent increase in basal insulin doses or basal insulin pump rate.
4. An error in basal or bolus insulin administration.
5. An error in diluting bolus insulin.
6. A recent increase in the amount of exercise.
7. A recent change in exercise type or intensity.
8. Improved insulin sensitivity due to unplanned physical activity or exercise.
9. Recent addition of another blood-sugar-lowering medication, e.g., metformin, pramlintide, SGLT2 inhibitor, or a GLP-1 agonist.
10. Overly aggressive insulin administration to correct high blood sugars including during an illness, a period of sleep deprivation, or women's menstrual cycles as discussed in Chapters 8 and 9.
11. Drinking alcohol can cause hypoglycemia due to suppressed liver glucose production as well as masking the symptoms of hypoglycemia which delays its treatment. Some alcoholic drinks are naturally high in carbohydrates (beer) while others are mixed with fruit juice or other sweet ingredients that can result in high blood sugars. See Chapter 8 for more details.

In general, erring on the side of a bit less insulin, rather than too much, is a guideline I advocate to avoid hypoglycemia especially when you're not confident of the insulin dose needed at any particular time. Having mildly elevated blood sugars from time to time is much safer than having hypoglycemia. As mentioned in Chapter 5, the use of a CGM equipped with a low glucose alarm and insulin pumps integrated with a CGM that can alarm and suspend insulin infusions in response to falling blood glucose are valuable safety features when sleeping, exercising, or driving a vehicle.

In summary, 1) hypoglycemia is dangerous and sometimes fatal, 2) hypoglycemia unawareness caused by exercise, sleep, alcohol, and the neuroadaptation to recurrent hypoglycemia increases the likelihood of hypoglycemia, 3) hypoglycemia unawareness due to recurrent hypoglycemia is reversible with 2–3 weeks of strict avoidance of hypoglycemia, 4) hypoglycemia unawareness can be prevented with continued avoidance of hypoglycemia, and 5) prevention of hypoglycemia should be our highest priority in the treatment of T1D even if that requires a higher-than-normal target blood glucose.

11 – Lipoproteins, CVD, Metformin & Symlin

"Necessity is the mother of invention."
Plato, Athenian philosopher.

"If Ali says a mosquito can pull a plow, don't argue, hitch it up."
Muhammad Ali, "The Greatest," professional boxer.

Low-Carbohydrate Diets & Elevations of LDL-C

This discussion will not address genetic causes of lipid abnormalities (familial hypercholesterolemia), but will only address isolated increases in total cholesterol (TC) and low-density lipoprotein cholesterol (LDL-C) that occur after adopting a LCD/VLCD. Whether the increase in TC and LDL-C represents an increased risk of CVD is unclear given that it has never been studied in those who follow a LCD/VLCD. We must understand that not all LDL particles are alike, but simply measuring LDL-C does not elucidate this fact. The LDL particles that most commonly lead to atherosclerosis and CVD are called small-dense LDL (sdLDL) particles. These particles typically form in persons with metabolic syndrome, insulin resistance, hyperinsulinemia, T2D, double diabetes, and hypertriglyceridemia [Julius, U, et al., 2007]. The LDL receptors in the liver have a reduced ability to remove sdLDL particles from the bloodstream due to a change in apolipoprotein B-100 (ApoB) conformation on the surface of sdLDL increasing their particle residence time [Thongtang, N, et al., 2017] and their tendency to penetrate the arterial wall where they become oxidized and glycated, forming atherosclerotic plaques [Ivanova,

EA, et al., 2017]. Conversely, in metabolically healthy individuals, large LDL particles are removed from the circulation by the LDL receptors in the liver, have a normal particle residence time, are not incorporated into the endothelium, and don't become oxidized or glycated or form atherosclerotic plaques. However, increases in both large and sdLDL particles can increase TC and LDL-C. This case-control study [Austin, MA, et al., 1988] measured LDL particle subclass patterns (pattern A, large LDL particle size vs. pattern B, sdLDL particle size measured by gel electrophoresis) in 109 cases of acute myocardial infarction (heart attack) and in 121 control subjects. The pattern B, sdLDL subclass pattern, was associated with a threefold increased risk of myocardial infarction. Interestingly, TC and LDL-C levels were not significantly related to myocardial infarction, or LDL subclass pattern, but the sdLDL subclass, pattern B, was associated with relative increases in serum triglycerides (TG), very low-density lipoprotein cholesterol (VLDL-C), intermediate-density lipoprotein cholesterol (IDL-C), and a reduction in HDL-C. VLDL and IDL particles are triglyceride-rich particles made in the liver and are the precursors of LDL particles. In those with metabolic syndrome, excess dietary carbohydrate is converted to TG by the liver via de novo lipogenesis and secreted as VLDL particles, ultimately becoming sdLDL particles. This is called atherogenic dyslipidemia of obesity, insulin resistance, and metabolic syndrome: the most prevalent lipid trait associated with CVD. Another study [St-Pierre, AC, et al., 2005] similarly concluded that pattern B, the sdLDL phenotype, confers an increased risk of CVD and that levels of large LDL are not associated with an increased risk of CVD in men.

Measuring LDL-C alone does not reveal the proportion of LDL particles that are small-dense vs. large and does not predict risk of CVD [Tsai, MY, et al., 2014]. We have two options to elucidate this important distinction.

We can get an advanced lipid profile that directly measures the LDL particle size and numbers in which low levels of sdLDL combined with low TG (< 100 mg/dl (< 1.1 mM)) and high HDL-C (> 40 mg/dl (> 1.0 mM) for men, or > 50 mg/dl (> 1.3 mM) for women), is referred to as pattern A (low CVD risk) or if you don't have access to advanced lipid profile testing, the next best option is to infer the presence of pattern A from low TG and VLDL-C and high HDL-C with the understanding that sdLDL can still be present in a minority of individuals. Two other indicators of low CVD risk include a zero CT coronary artery calcium score and hsCRP (a marker of chronic inflammation, normal is < 1.0 mg/L).

In the majority of those implementing a LCD, lipid markers improve compared to a LFHCD even without weight loss [Feinman, RD, 2006, Musunuru, K, 2010, Volek, JS, et al., 2005]. This one year clinical trial [Cicero, AFG, et al., 2015] of a ketogenic VLCD showed multiple improvements in body composition, blood pressure, blood glucose (fasting and HbA1c), and lipid parameters. The LDL-C significantly improved from baseline to 3 months (−19.5 ± 16.9 mg/dl) with no change after 1 year of observation. A similar trend was observed for TG (−23.4 ± 30.2 mg/dl), while HDL-C improved from baseline to 4 weeks (+1.8 ± 5.6 mg/dl), and even more after 12 months (+3.5 ± 3.3 mg/dl). This study [Forsythe, CE, et al., 2008] found that a VLCD resulted in profound and favorable changes in serum fatty acid composition and reduced markers of chronic inflammation compared to a LFHCD. The ketogenic VLCD reduces TG, oxidized and glycated sdLDL particles, and serum insulin levels, while increasing HDL-C, consistent with reduced risk for CVD [Volek, JS, et al., 2008].

Lipoprotein levels can simply be a reflection of one's diet and daily energy expenditure. The purpose of VLDL, IDL, and LDL in metabolically healthy individuals is to transport energy in the form of TG from the liver and fat cells to cells throughout the body. This study [Sävendahl, L, et al., 1999] found that LDL-C and ApoB increased by ≈ 66% in healthy, nonobese subjects after a 7-day fast. Because fat is the primary source of energy during fasting, after a VLDL particle has delivered its TG content to the body's cells, it becomes an IDL, then an LDL particle, and can increase the LDL-C in the blood as this study demonstrated. It is certainly conceivable that by following a VLCD where fat is the primary fuel, especially in those who exercise prodigiously, that elevations in LDL-C and ApoB are appropriate for the purpose of transporting TG rather than being a reflection of increased sdLDL particles and CVD risk. These factors should be taken into account when deciding how to respond to isolated increases in TC and LDL-C after adopting a LCD/VLCD.

Total dietary fat and SFA in a LCD will increase large particle LDL and may account for the increase in LDL-C after starting a LCD/VLCD [Krauss, RM, et al., 2006, Bergeron, N, et al., 2019]. If you would like to reduce your LDL-C even though the large LDL particles are not associated with an increased CVD risk, you can simply replace SFA from meat, pork, lamb, poultry, animal fat (lard, tallow, suet), butter, cheese, and coconut oil with MUFA from nuts, seeds, fish, and the oils of macadamia nuts, avocados, and olives. If this maneuver does not decrease LDL-C to a 'satisfactory level,' you will ultimately have to decide whether to 1) continue your LCD with emphasis on MUFA, 2) incorporate more carbohydrates into your diet and hope your glycemic control does not deteriorate, or 3) take a statin medication which is generally recommended to those with diabetes regardless of their lipoprotein levels. This study [Mitchell, JD, et al., 2018] examined the benefit of statin therapy in preventing a first major adverse cardiovascular event (MACE) based on the coronary artery calcium score (CAC) of 13,644 patients (mean age 50 years; 71% men) who were followed for a median of 9.4 years. Statin therapy was associated with reduced risk of MACE in patients with CAC > 0, but not in patients with a zero CAC. The effect of statin use on MACE was significantly related to the severity of CAC, with the number needed to treat (NNT) to prevent one initial MACE outcome over 10 years ranging from 100 (for a CAC of 1–100) to 12 (for a CAC > 100). The authors concluded that amongst the study participants, increasing severity of CAC was associated with increased benefit from statin treatment for the prevention of MACE, with greatest benefit in patients with CAC > 100. You should discuss this issue with your physician as part of your decision-making process. Those who choose to take a statin should consider supplementing with coenzyme Q10 [Deichmann, R, et al., 2010].

Reducing Cardiovascular Disease Risk in Those With T1D

Since CVD is the number one cause of death in those with T1D, if we can identify and correct all of the known modifiable risk factors for CVD, we can reduce our risk of developing CVD and extend our health-span and lifespan. Risk factors for CVD in those with T1D ordered from most to least impactful are: 1) poor glycemic control, 2) high blood pressure, 3) microalbuminuria (indicative of diabetic nephropathy), 4) systemic inflammation, 5) cigarette smoking, 6) insulin resistance, and 7) high LDL-C (see above) [see Table 2, de Ferranti, SD, et al., 2014]. The strategies in this book address all of these risk factors directly or indirectly. The main theme of this book, normalizing blood sugars, addresses the #1 risk factor for CVD. High blood pressure often results from insulin resistance and metabolic syndrome which can be resolved with a LCD, lower insulin doses, improved body composition, and exercise. Microalbuminuria is a manifestation of diabetic nephropathy due to poor glycemic control, but is likely reversible with normalization of blood sugars in the setting of normal kidney function. You should obviously stop smoking if you are currently doing so. Additional factors that adversely affect glycemic control and lead to chronic inflammation and numerous chronic diseases including CVD are: 1) dietary sugar, refined carbohydrates, and vegetable oils found in processed foods, 2) visceral obesity [Ormazabal, V, et al., 2018], 3) sedentary lifestyle [Parsons, TJ, et al., 2017], 4) poor sleep hygiene [Mullington, JM, et al., 2010], 5) chronic stress [Liu, Y, et al., 2017], 6) smoking [McEvoy, JW, et al., 2015], 7) alcohol [Osna, NA, 2010], and 8) inadequate sunlight exposure [Hoel, GD, et al., 2016]. A LCD/VLCD reduces markers of systemic inflammation [Forsythe, CE, et al., 2008] and improves visceral obesity [Miyashita, Y, et al., 2004]. Poor glycemic control, high glycemic variation, and high insulin doses directly impact complication-prone cells in the eye, kidney, and nerves via production of reactive oxygen species and chronic systemic inflammation. When a LCD/VLCD along with the other strategies in this book improve glycemic control and variation, reduce chronic inflammation and excess body fat, and improve insulin sensitivity with lower exogenous insulin doses, we would expect the risk of CVD to be lower as well.

Is There Evidence That a LCD Prevents CVD?

A RCT should be done to test the efficacy of a LCD/VLCD in normalizing blood sugars and preventing or reversing long-term diabetic complications and CVD. It may be a long time before such a RCT is completed, but in the meantime, I don't think it is prudent to tolerate poor glycemic control. Thus, I have chosen to extrapolate from the results of the DCCT and hypothesize that normal blood sugars will improve and/or prevent diabetic complications including CVD. The DCCT/EDIC study

[The DCCT/EDIC Study Research Group, 2005], followed the 1,441 patients from the DCCT for 17 years and found that "46 CVD events occurred in 31 patients who had received intensive [insulin] treatment in the DCCT, as compared with 98 events in 52 patients who had received conventional [insulin] treatment." The authors concluded that "Intensive diabetes therapy has long-term beneficial effects on the risk of CVD in patients with T1D." While I admit my approach is untested, the current approach to treating T1D has resulted in an average HbA1c among 16,061 persons in the T1D Exchange Clinic Registry of 8.4% as of 2014 [Miller, KM, et al., 2015]. I will let these results and the diabetic complications, CVD, and 11–13 year reduction in lifespan [Livingstone, SJ, et al., 2015] that these persons must endure speak for the effectiveness of the current approach to treating T1D.

Metformin

Metformin is the most prescribed diabetes medication worldwide. Although it is primarily used for T2D, metformin has been studied and used for T1D to improve insulin resistance, assist in weight loss, and reduce insulin dosage in those with T1D and double diabetes. It is a very safe medication with minor and reversible gastrointestinal side-effects including nausea, diarrhea, and abdominal discomfort which can largely be avoided by starting with a low dose and increasing the dose slowly over time. For example, metformin can be started at 500 mg/day and increased by 500 mg/day every 2–3 weeks as tolerated up to the maximum dose: 2,000–2,550 mg/day. Immediate-release metformin comes in 500 mg, 850 mg, and 1,000 mg tablets. Extended-release metformin comes in 500 mg and 750 mg tablets and can sometimes mitigate the gastrointestinal side-effects of immediate-release metformin. Metformin should be taken before meals to attenuate the rise in post-meal blood glucose. I suggest not doubling-up with a missed dose since it might increase the likelihood of hypoglycemia.

Metformin improves insulin sensitivity by stimulating glucose uptake primarily in skeletal muscle. It also increases the binding of insulin to its receptor and decreases glucose production by the liver [Madiraju, AK, et al., 2014]. This helps to suppress post-meal liver glucose production due to amino-acid stimulated α-cell glucagon secretion. Thus, the combination of a LCD/VLCD, which reduces dietary carbohydrate intake, and metformin, which reduces the glucose-raising effect of the protein in a meal, results in improved post-meal blood sugars while using smaller BID. This meta-analysis [Liu, C, et al., 2015] of metformin use in T1D included eight RCT. Metformin was associated with a reduction in TDID (1.36 IU/day) and bodyweight (2.41 kg), but an increase in gastrointestinal side-effects compared with placebo. No significant difference was found between the metformin and placebo groups in HbA1c, fasting blood glucose, plasma triglycerides, risk of severe hypoglycemia, or DKA.

Despite not being overweight or insulin resistant, I decided to try metformin in December 2017. My TDID decreased by $\approx$ 10% with no change in hypoglycemia, mean blood glucose, or bodyweight and no adverse side-effects. On occasions when I forgot to take a dose of metformin, I noted a higher-than-usual post-meal blood sugar consistent with its continued effectiveness. I currently take 1,000 mg with breakfast and dinner. Because metformin is such an inexpensive medication, taking it is a cost-saving measure due to the reduction in TDID. The primary reason I will continue taking metformin is to reduce my lifetime exposure to insulin which I believe reduces the likelihood of a host of chronic diseases and therefore may improve my health-span and lifespan.

I wanted to make you aware of three studies recently published regarding the attenuation of the beneficial effects of exercise in subjects taking metformin. These subjects were either healthy or had prediabetes, but none had T1D, meaning none of these studies may be applicable to those with T1D. The first was a RCT [Walton, RG, et al., 2019] that measured the effect of metformin (n = 46) vs. placebo (n = 48) on muscle hypertrophy and strength in healthy men and women, age ≥ 65 years, in response to progressive resistance exercise training (PRT). The authors concluded that "Although responses to PRT varied, placebo gained more lean body mass (p = 0.003) and thigh muscle mass (p < 0.001) than metformin. CT scan showed that increases in thigh muscle area (p = 0.005) and density (p = 0.020) were greater in placebo versus metformin." In a smaller clinical trial [Malin, SK, et al., 2012], "For 12 weeks, men and women with prediabetes were assigned to the following groups: placebo (P), 2,000 mg/day metformin (M), exercise training with placebo (EP), or exercise training with metformin (EM) (n = 8 per group). Before and after the intervention, insulin sensitivity was measured by euglycemic hyperinsulinemic clamp. Insulin sensitivity was considerably higher after 12 weeks of exercise training and/or metformin in men and women with prediabetes. Subtle differences [i.e., statistically nonsignificant] among condition means [i.e., averages] suggest that adding metformin blunted the full effect of exercise training." A third study [Konopka, AR, et al., 2019], "tested the hypothesis that metformin diminishes the improvement in insulin sensitivity and cardiorespiratory fitness after aerobic exercise training (AET) by inhibiting skeletal muscle mitochondrial respiration and protein synthesis in older adults (62 ± 1 years). In a double-blinded fashion, participants were randomized to placebo (n = 26) or metformin (n = 27) treatment during 12 weeks of AET. Independent of treatment, AET decreased fat mass, HbA1c, fasting plasma insulin, 24-hr ambulant mean glucose, and glycemic variability. However, metformin attenuated the increase in whole-body insulin sensitivity and VO_2max after AET. In the metformin group, there was no overall change in whole-body insulin sensitivity after AET due to positive and negative responders. Metformin also abrogated the exercise-mediated increase in skeletal muscle mitochondrial respiration."

The decision to take any medication involves weighing benefits vs. risks. I have a keen interest in physical training and retention of muscle mass as I age. I also want to limit my lifetime exposure to insulin. As you know, I have decided to take metformin despite the findings of the studies presented above. A closer examination of the data in the studies made me less concerned about their findings. By examining Figures 2 and 4 in the first study, you will see what the authors meant by, "Although responses to PRT varied, ..." Upon my examination, there was no clear-cut difference between the change in muscle mass, area, or density in response to PRT in those taking placebo vs. metformin. Similarly, my examination of Figure 1 in the third study, showed no clear-cut difference between the whole-body insulin sensitivity and VO_2max in response to AET in those taking placebo vs. metformin. Additionally, the authors point out that, "However, metformin did not inhibit other AET improvements, including telomere elongation, fasting insulin, 24-hr mean glucose, and body composition."

Finally, it has been reported that 30% of patients receiving long-term metformin treatment experienced malabsorption of vitamin B12, with a decrease in serum vitamin B12 concentration of 14% to 30% [Ting, RZ, et al., 2006]. Dose and duration of metformin use were the strongest predictors of developing vitamin B12 deficiency. This systematic review [Liu, Q, et al., 2014] of six RCT examining vitamin B12 status in individuals taking metformin vs. placebo or rosiglitazone (an oral medication for T2D) concluded that "The reduction of vitamin B12 may be induced by metformin in a dose dependent manner." Additionally, those with T1D are at increased risk for autoimmune pernicious anemia and celiac disease, both of which interfere with vitamin B12 absorption [Kibirige, D, et al., 2013]. Thus, if you choose to take metformin you should ensure your vitamin B12 intake is more than adequate even if that requires supplementation and you might also consider checking a vitamin B12 level several months after starting metformin to make sure your level is in the normal range.

Pramlintide (Symlin)

Pramlintide (Symlin) is a pharmaceutical form of the hormone, amylin, that is normally cosecreted with insulin by the β-cells in the pancreas. Amylin has three known effects: 1) it suppresses α-cell glucagon secretion, 2) it slows the rate of stomach emptying which delays the absorption of nutrients, and 3) it suppresses appetite. Because amylin secretion is virtually absent in T1D, 1) liver glucose production is increased after meals due to the lack of suppression of α-cell glucagon secretion, 2) the stomach empties more quickly increasing the rate of rise in post-meal blood sugar particularly when consuming carbohydrates, and 3) can increase appetite and food consumption, all of which raise blood sugar. As you have learned, a LCD reduces the rate of rise in post-meal blood sugar and reduces appetite which may mitigate the loss of amylin secretion, especially if metformin is utilized to suppress liver glucose production.

Pramlintide (Symlin) is an injectable medication that comes in a 1.5 mL or 2.7 mL disposable multidose SymlinPen® 60 pen-injector containing 1000 mcg/ml of pramlintide. It is used only prior to meals to reduce the post-meal blood sugar excursion. An initial 50% reduction in the mealtime insulin dose is generally recommended to avoid hypoglycemia. Nausea is the main side-effect of pramlintide (Symlin) which can be reduced by starting with the lowest dose and slowly increasing it over time. Interestingly, this study found that although post-meal plasma glucagon excursions were lower after pramlintide (Symlin) compared to placebo in 12 patients with T1D, endogenous glucose production was no different suggesting that delayed gastric emptying and slowed carbohydrate absorption were the main mechanisms attenuating the rise in post-meal blood glucose [Hinshaw, L, et al., 2016]. This was a small study, but if it is correct, one would predict pramlintide (Symlin) would be less effective in those consuming a LCD. This paper [Lee, NJ, et al., 2010] reviewed the literature and found three RCT comparing pramlintide (Symlin) to placebo in T1D patients for 6–12 months. One trial found no improvement in HbA1c in T1D patients using intensive insulin therapy, while two trials found HbA1c improved by 0.2–0.3% in T1D patients using conventional insulin therapy. Changes in TDID were small for both pramlintide (range, –12% to +2.3%) and placebo (range, 0.0% to +10.3%). Weight loss was consistently greater in patients using pramlintide (range of mean change across 3 trials, –0.4 kg to –1.3 kg) compared to placebo (+0.8 kg to +1.2 kg).

I have never prescribed pramlintide (Symlin) nor used it myself, but I have spoken with a few T1D patients who have benefitted from it. Your physician can help you to safely utilize this medication should you decide to try it. Now that Symlin is off-patent, generic versions of pramlintide may be more reasonably priced.

12 – Improving Body Composition

"If it's important, you'll find a way. If it's not, you'll find an excuse."
Ryan Blair, Author of *Nothing to Lose, Everything to Gain*.

"Only I can change my life. No one can do it for me."
Carol Burnett, an American actress, comedian, singer, and writer.

"Whether you think you can, or you think you can't — you're right."
Henry Ford, the founder of Ford Motor Company.

"Failure is not an option."
Gene Kranz, NASA Flight Director of the Gemini and Apollo programs.

Although the process of designing a LCD/VLCD to lose excess body fat was covered in Chapter 4, this chapter provides some additional information and suggestions on this important topic.

Extent and Causes of Excess Body Fat in T1D

There are numerous causes of excess body fat and its resolution does not have a single simple solution. The U.S. SEARCH for Diabetes in Youth study [Liu, LL, et al., 2010] found that 22.1% of youths with T1D were overweight and 12.6% were obese. The prevalence of overweight and obesity at onset of insulin-dependent diabetes among 189 children in The Children's Hospital of Pittsburgh almost tripled from 12.6% to 36.8% between the time periods 1979–1989 and 1990–1998 [Libman, IM, et al., 2003]. In those with T1D, the anabolic effects of insulin "… are enhanced by exogenous insulin administration, since exogenous insulin imperfectly mimics endogenous secretion. While endogenous insulin has its first pass to the liver through the portal vein to suppress gluconeogenesis, exogenous insulin circulates systemically first and disproportionately affects muscle and adipose in comparison to the liver" [Mottalib, A, et al., 2017]. My opinion is that the LFHCD is the primary culprit, not intensive insulin therapy.

The hypothalamus in the brain plays an important role in the control of food intake. The lateral nuclei of the hypothalamus serve as a feeding center, whereas, the ventromedial nuclei of the hypothalamus serve as a major satiety center. The hypothalamus receives 1) neural signals from the gastrointestinal tract that provide sensory information about stomach filling; 2) chemical signals from nutrients in the blood (glucose, amino acids, and fatty acids) that increase satiety; 3) signals from gastrointestinal hormones, cholecystokinin (CCK) and peptide YY, that increase satiety, and ghrelin, that increases hunger; 4) signals from the fat cell hormone, leptin, that increases satiety; 5) signals from insulin that increases satiety; and 6) signals from the cerebral cortex, sight, smell, and taste, that influence feeding behavior. Interestingly, while insulin increases satiety in the brain, the removal of nutrients from the bloodstream by insulin can subsequently increase hunger.

Processed foods, now ubiquitous in Western societies, were introduced in the 1960s after which the pandemics of obesity, insulin resistance, and T2D became apparent. Processed foods are specifically designed to be convenient and addictive and are also highly profitable for the food industry by using ingredients (corn, wheat, sugar, and soybeans) subsidized by the U.S. government. Processed foods are typically lower in protein and high in sugar, refined carbohydrates, and/or vegetable oils in varying proportions. This combination of macronutrients stimulates the reward center in our brains to increase appetite and encourage us to repeatedly eat excessive amounts of these foods in the short- and long-term [DiFeliceantonio, AG, et al., 2018]. In vulnerable individuals, consumption of palatable foods can enhance the reinforcing value of food and weaken the inhibitory control circuits [Volkow, ND, et al., 2011]. This is illustrated by the top 10 sources of calories in the U.S. diet [What Americans Eat, 2010]: 1) grain-based desserts (cakes, cookies, donuts, pies, crisps, cobblers, and granola bars), 2) yeast breads, 3) chicken and chicken-mixed dishes, 4) soda, energy drinks, and sports drinks, 5) pizza, 6) alcoholic beverages, 7) pasta and pasta dishes, 8) mexican mixed dishes, 9) beef and beef-mixed dishes, and 10) dairy desserts.

This study [Hall, KD, et al., 2019] found that "... a diet with a large proportion of ultra-processed food increases energy intake and leads to weight gain." Interestingly, both fasting insulin and C-peptide levels were significantly reduced on the unprocessed-food diet compared to baseline levels. A similar explanation for the origin of our obesity, diabetes, and chronic disease pandemics is the protein leverage hypothesis [Simpson, SJ, et al., 2005] which contends that humans will continue to eat until they obtain an adequate dietary protein intake. The majority of modern human populations eating natural whole foods typically consume about 15% of total calories from protein. But people who rely on processed foods which are lower in protein and higher in carbohydrate and fat compared to whole foods, will consume these foods until they reach their bodies' protein needs. This requires that they consume excess calories just to meet their protein requirements, thus becoming obese or otherwise metabolically disturbed. And a third related explanation for the origin of our obesity, diabetes, and chronic disease pandemics is the carbohydrate-insulin model of obesity [Ludwig, DS, et al., 2018] which posits that "recent increases in the consumption of processed, high–glycemic-load carbohydrates produce hormonal changes that promote calorie deposition in adipose tissue, exacerbate hunger, and lower energy expenditure." In this model, overeating is the result, not the cause, of body fat accumulation. Note that all three of the above hypotheses proposed to explain the current obesity, diabetes, and chronic disease pandemics identify processed foods as the probable culprit and involve higher levels of insulin to deal with the refined carbohydrates and sugar. I have presented much evidence that a whole, unprocessed, low glycemic index/load LCD/VLCD is one effective strategy for improving body composition and blood sugars that also requires lower insulin doses. In summary, overweight and obesity is a complex disease with many contributing genetic, epigenetic [Thaker, VV, 2017], hormonal, environmental, and dietary factors. Although we can't change our genes, we can change which genes are expressed (epigenetic) and improve the other three factors that lead to overweight and obesity.

The Consequences of Excess Body Fat in T1D

The consequences of overweight and obesity in those with T1D are the same as for the general population, namely a higher incidence of insulin resistance, metabolic syndrome, double diabetes, and a multitude of chronic diseases including NAFLD [Regnell, SE, et al., 2011], CVD, and cancer. Sugar and high-fructose corn syrup (HFCS), particularly in beverages, likely play a causative role in both obesity and cancer. This study [Goncalves, MD, et al., 2019] in mice prone to develop intestinal polyps found that even moderate amounts of HFCS (equivalent to 12 oz of Coca-Cola per day in humans) caused a substantial increase in intestinal tumor size and tumor grade prior to the development of obesity and

metabolic syndrome. Metabolic syndrome in those with T1D is present if two of the following four criteria are met:
1. Abdominal obesity: waist circumference > 40 inches (102 cm) for men, or > 35 inches (90 cm) for women.
2. Blood pressure > 130/85 mmHg.
3. Fasting serum triglyceride (TG) > 150 mg/dl (> 1.7 mM).
4. Fasting high-density lipoprotein cholesterol (HDL-C) < 40 mg/dl (< 1.0 mM) for men, or < 50 mg/dl (< 1.3 mM) for women.

Although high LDL-C is not part of the criteria for metabolic syndrome: small-dense LDL (sdLDL) particles are often increased (referred to as Pattern B). This atherogenic dyslipidemia of metabolic syndrome, even prior to the development of diabetes, has been documented to be associated with an increased risk of CVD. Beginning in the 1960s, Drs. Albrink, Man, Kuo, Ahrens, and Reaven were pioneers in unraveling the link between excess dietary starch, and particularly sugar, in the development of hypertriglyceridemia, especially in those with insulin resistance, and its association with CVD [Ahrens, EH, et al., 1961, Albrink, MJ, et al., 1961, Kuo, PT, et al., 1965, Reaven, GM, et al., 1967].

Our body's ability to store dietary carbohydrate for future use is quite limited relative to our ability to store dietary fat. A 70 kg adult male has the ability to store about 400 kcal as liver glycogen, 24,000 kcal as muscle glycogen, and 110,000 kcal as fat [Cahill, GF, et al., 2003]. Excess dietary carbohydrate that can't be used immediately for energy will be stored as liver and muscle glycogen and/or converted to triglycerides in liver and/or fat cells via de novo lipogenesis. A high-carbohydrate diet, especially one with sugar and fructose, increases de novo lipogenesis in the liver and increases VLDL and triglycerides in the blood. A metabolically-healthy person can safely store triglycerides in subcutaneous fat cells, but insulin-resistant individuals will tend to store triglycerides in their abdominal organs, called visceral fat, because the subcutaneous fat cells are resistant to taking up additional triglycerides. This can cause NAFLD [Jensen, T, et al., 2018] and eventually liver cirrhosis which now exceeds alcoholic cirrhosis as the leading cause of liver failure and transplantation. The deposition of fat in the pancreas can cause insulin resistance and β-cell dysfunction leading to T2D [Lu, T, et al. 2019] and presumably double diabetes. This study [Merger, SR, et al., 2016] found that 25.5% of 31,119 persons with T1D met the criteria for metabolic syndrome. Because double diabetes is associated with an increase in diabetic complications independent of blood sugar control, reversing this condition will improve the life and longevity of those with T1D. A LCD/VLCD has been shown to improve or reverse the metabolic syndrome [Athinarayanan, SJ, et al., 2019, Hyde, PN, et al., 2019]. Excess body fat contributes to insulin resistance and causes hypertrophic fat cells to secrete inflammatory adipokines including high sensitivity C-reactive protein (hsCRP), tumor necrosis factor-α (TNFα), interleukin-6 (IL-6), resistin, and plasminogen activator inhibitor-1 (PAI-1), and reduce secretion of beneficial adipokines like adiponectin. These inflammatory adipokines contribute to the development of metabolic syndrome, double diabetes, and CVD [Haffner, SM, 2006].

Losing Body Fat While Achieving Normal Blood Sugars

While it is clear that the types of food one consumes is an important determinant of gaining or losing body fat [Johnson, RJ, et al., 2017, Ludwig, DS, et al., 2018], the total amount (calories) of food also matters. Given that it is possible to eat beyond one's satiety signals on a LCD, quantitating food intake can help with losing body fat as well as predicting BID to normalize blood sugars. The quantity of food eaten (calories) can be gradually reduced in small steps over time to shed body fat. Caloric intake can be estimated using cronometer.com as discussed in Chapter 4. By tracking the progress of your body fat loss, you can infer whether or not your food/caloric intake is appropriate and adjust it accordingly. A common misconception about the formulation of a LCD, and particularly that of a ketogenic VLCD, is that dietary fat intake should be specifically increased. Often the term, low-carbohydrate high-fat (LCHF) diet is used to describe a VLCD. Others have suggested that LCHF should instead stand for 'low-carbohydrate healthful-fat,' with which I agree. Specifically trying increase one's dietary fat intake is fine for those with a higher daily caloric expenditure, but can certainly thwart one's efforts to lose body fat. Since dietary protein and carbohydrate are essentially fixed on a LCD/VLCD, dietary fat is the only remaining macronutrient that can be decreased to lose body fat. Thus, to lose body fat while maintaining normal blood sugars with T1D, you need to 1) follow a LCD/VLCD with emphasis on dietary protein intake as shown in Table 4.11, 2) reduce dietary fat intake in 22 g/day steps while avoiding hunger, and 3) quantitate food intake at each meal to be able to predict BID. Avoiding hunger is important in this process since as Robert Atkins, MD said in his book, *The Atkins New Diet Revolution*, "Although many people can tolerate hunger for a while, very few can tolerate it for a lifetime." The control of hunger is one of the chief advantages of adopting a higher-protein LCD during and after fat loss [Gibson, AA, et al., 2015]. Increasing the percentage of calories from dietary protein is beneficial due to increased satiety, the larger thermic effect of protein, and maintenance or accretion of lean muscle mass [Paddon-Jones, D, et al., 2008]. The thermic effect of food (TEF) represents a transient increase in energy expenditure attributable to nutrient processing (i.e. digestion, absorption, transport, metabolism and storage of nutrients) and is expressed as a percentage increase in energy expenditure above the basal metabolic rate.

TEF is highest for protein (≈ 15–30%), followed by carbohydrate (≈ 5–10%) and fat (≈ 0–3%).

Ideally, we would like the majority of weight loss to come from fat stores and minimize the amount of muscle mass loss since muscle is the primary source of glucose consumption. Muscle mass during weight loss is preserved when the degree of caloric restriction and the rate of weight loss is more modest [Garthe, I, et al., 2011]. It is also established that both aerobic and resistance exercise help to preserve or increase fat-free mass during weight loss [Chaston, TB, et al., 2007, Phillips, SM, 2014].

Quantitating food intake helps to appropriately reduce food intake without depending on your visual estimation of meal size. Quantitating food intake at each meal can be accomplished by: 1) counting pre-portioned foodstuffs, e.g., four large eggs or two strips of bacon, 2) weighing your food using a kitchen scale, 3) dividing pre-measured portions by eye, e.g., cutting an 8 oz uniformly-shaped block of cheese into eight 1-ounce pieces, and, 4) after some experience having utilized a kitchen scale, by eye alone. I use the first three methods when eating at home and the last method when traveling or eating in restaurants. Kitchen scales are battery operated and can be brought to a restaurant, although this may be socially awkward for some. A kitchen scale is also useful at home when weighing ingredients to make a recipe. I use my kitchen scale to weigh the ingredients of my keto chocolate mousse dessert which I make once a week. I divide the total weight of the recipe by 21 (7 days × 3 meals/day) and use my kitchen scale to weigh the portion I eat at each meal. By using these quantification methods, my meals do not vary from day to day, my BID is more predictable, my post-meal blood glucose stays in my target range 70–130 mg/dl (3.9–7.2 mM) most of the time, and my bodyweight remains at my goal, 73 kg. The quantity of dietary fat can be reduced by a modest 22 g/day and periodically (≈ 3–4 weeks) adjusted as needed to improve body composition. This 3–4 week period allows time to both decrease insulin doses to maintain normal blood sugars and to assess your response to the change in food quantity in terms of how you feel and your change in body composition. Body composition can be assessed by your appearance in the mirror, waist circumference, and/or bodyweight. Remember bodyweight is influenced by several other factors including muscle mass, water weight, and bowel movements, such that assessing body fat loss with bodyweight alone is not necessarily reliable. A waist-to-height ratio of < 0.5 correlates with metabolic health and is a useful goal to aim for as well [Ferreira-Hermosillo, A, et al., 2014]. The amount of decrease in caloric intake and the frequency of the reductions I mentioned above may not be perfect for everyone, but can serve as a starting point to be adjusted based on your own experience.

There are an increasing number of convenient 'keto' food products and snacks appearing in stores and online. I would caution you from thinking that if 'keto' is on the label, it means it is a good thing for you to eat. Processed 'keto' foods are still processed foods. You should examine the ingredient list carefully to decide whether or not you want to consume it, especially on a regular basis. Keto-processed foods often contain ingredients you may not want to eat including nut flours, preservatives, emulsifiers, artificial sweeteners, colors, flavors, and vegetable oils. These ingredients are added to processed foods to increase their shelf life, prevent fats from separating, and make them appear and taste more appealing. They typically will emphasize the net carb count on the label, rather than total carbohydrates which masks the sugar-alcohol content. In terms of controlling blood sugars, restricting total carbohydrates is the most effective strategy. These foods may temporarily help some with the transition to low-carbohydrate whole foods, but I would avoid thinking they are appropriate for the long-term. For those with T1D, consuming snacks between meals presents a special challenge with blood sugar regulation. Including one or more snacks in your daily food plan may be okay if: 1) you do not need to inject extra insulin to prevent the snack from increasing your blood sugar, 2) the ingredients are healthful, 3) you are already at goal weight, and 4) you consume the same snack (or same macronutrients), at the same time, everyday.

Physical Activity Facilitates Body Fat Loss

This review article [Mottalib, A, et al., 2017] states that, "Although weight loss can be achieved with only restriction of energy intake, increasing physical activity and incorporating exercise training into a weight loss plan lead to greater loss of fat mass and preservation of lean muscle mass compared to energy restriction alone [Chimen, M, et al., 2012, Miller, CT, et al., 2013]. Additionally, there are metabolic benefits to partaking in physical activity for weight loss. In patients with T1D, physical activity has been shown to decrease CVD risk and mortality [Washburn, RA, et al. 2014], in addition to improving endothelial function and lipid profiles [Fuchsjäger-Mayrl, G, et al., 2002]." Physical activity promotes secretion of beneficial myokines such as myostatin, irisin, interleukin-6 and -15, brain-derived neurotrophic factor (BDNF), and myonectin, to name a few [Lee, JH, et al., 2019]. Myokines are cytokines synthesized and released by muscle cells during muscular contractions. They favorably regulate metabolism in muscle, fat tissue, liver, and brain. Exercise, a ketogenic VLCD, cold-water immersion, and acclimation to over-night temperature reduction, promote the conversion of white fat cells to either brown or beige fat cells [Lee, P, et al., 2014]. These interventions appear to increase energy utilization allowing for more effective body fat loss [Leal, LG, et al., 2018]. Beige and brown fat cells contain numerous mitochondria giving them the brown coloration. These mitochondria produce heat, consuming energy in the process, via an uncoupling of the proton gradient. While cold-water immersion can promote the conversion of white fat to beige fat, when done soon after exercise, may attenuate the benefits of exercise training [Méline, T, 2017]. "Exercise remains one of the best ways to stimulate mitochondrial biogenesis and is likely key to long-term success for any weight-loss program" [Johnson, RJ, et al., 2017].

Compliance & Consistency

Constructing a well-formulated LCD with modest caloric reduction progressively over time to avoid hunger while shedding body fat slowly and supporting muscle mass with resistance exercise and adequate dietary protein intake are important strategies for weight loss success. "An emerging body of evidence suggests that a higher level of adherence to a diet, regardless of the type of diet, is an important factor in weight loss success over the short and long term. Key strategies to improve adherence include designing dietary weight loss interventions (such as ketogenic diets) that help to control the increased drive to eat that accompanies weight loss, tailoring dietary interventions to a person's dietary preferences (and nutritional requirements), and promoting self-monitoring [i.e., quantification] of food intake" [Gibson, AA, et al., 2017]. Cheating on a diet prevents or delays attaining one's weight and blood sugar goals. If having an improved body composition and normal blood sugars are important to you, then I'm sure you'll find a way to stick with your new lifestyle.

This is a summary of the steps needed to lose body fat while achieving normal blood sugars:

1. Enter all the foods you are currently eating in a day into cronometer.com and subtract 200 kcal/day as a starting caloric intake or choose a goal bodyweight and suggested caloric intake as discussed in Chapter 4. The reduction in caloric intake will come almost exclusively from dietary fat because dietary carbohydrate is already restricted by design and dietary protein is set to preserve lean body mass during the weight-loss process (Table 4.11).

2. Use cronometer.com, or another resource, to design specific meals as directed in Chapter 4. This means you will have a target number of macronutrient grams, i.e., dietary protein, carbohydrate, and fat for each meal and will design your meals to match these goals (e.g., see Table 4.12). Repeating the same meal from day to day is the most effective way to achieve normal blood sugars, while the second most effective approach is to vary the food, but keep the macronutrient amounts (in grams) for any given meal constant from day to day.

3. Stick with the same meals (or macronutrients) each day for ≈ 3–4 weeks to allow time to both adjust insulin doses to maintain or reestablish normal blood sugars and to assess your response to the change in terms of how you feel and your body composition as assessed by appearance, waist circumference, and/or bodyweight.

4. If you are feeling well and your blood sugars are close to your target, but you are not seeing any progress with your body composition, then decrease your fat intake by 22 g/day.

5. If you are having symptoms of insufficient caloric intake, increase your fat intake by 22 g/day.

6. If you were in the habit of consuming a large amount of food, then it may require numerous 22 g/day dietary fat reductions to shed body fat. Be patient. You did not gain the excess body fat in a short time and there is rarely a need to lose it in a short time. If you do need to

remove body fat in a short time due to a severe medical condition, you should be seeing a physician with experience in obesity medicine.

7. Starting a daily exercise program can help facilitate weight loss while maintaining lean muscle mass. Walking is always a good place to start. Resistance exercise is the most effective means to build and maintain muscle mass and burn glucose and calories the entire day. That said, the best exercise is the one you will do everyday. Even though exercise produces modest weight loss, the health benefits of exercise extend far beyond weight loss. As you shed body fat, you will feel like doing more exercise. Increase the amount, duration, or intensity of exercise gradually over time as you feel able to.

8. Some who are overweight, in addition to the factors mentioned above, eat for reasons other than appropriate hunger. In some cases, emotional eating relieves different kinds of stress. Others eat due to the brain signals created by processed foods rather than the body's need for nutrients. Some eat as a form of entertainment or simply do not have other activities to do that they enjoy. Changing to a LCD, absent of processed foods, may be enough to solve these problems, while others may benefit from an obesity medicine consultation.

Obesity Medicine Physician Consultation

While it is true that one must create a caloric deficit to lose body fat, reducing caloric intake, in some cases, can result in a compensatory decrease in caloric expenditure, and conversely, increasing physical activity can result in a desire to eat more food, which if not provided, can cause hunger. Hormones including insulin, estrogen, testosterone, leptin, and ghrelin can affect one's ability to lose body fat. Thus in some persons with T1D, adopting a well-formulated LCD/VLCD with reduced insulin doses, confirming compliance with it, quantitating food intake, reducing dietary fat intake in modest steps, and increasing physical activity may not be enough to reach one's body composition goal. An obesity medicine physician may be able to uncover a cause(s) for your inability to achieve your goal body composition and formulate a treatment plan. They will review your medications and screen for medical conditions that can interfere with weight loss including sleep apnea, Cushing's disease, and hypothyroidism, and discuss other available options for success.

13 – Ketosis & Diabetic Ketoacidosis

"If everyone is thinking alike, then somebody isn't thinking."
General George S. Patton, United States Army.

"Ninety-nine percent of the failures come from people who have the habit of making excuses."
George Washington Carver, American agricultural scientist and inventor.

Ketones and Nutritional Ketosis

Nutritional ketosis is the normal physiological state that results from consuming a VLCD (≤ 50 grams carbohydrate/day). After beginning a VLCD, the body undergoes keto-adaptation, increasing the enzymes needed to produce, transport (via monocarboxylate transporters), and utilize ketone bodies and fatty acids more efficiently [Volek, JS, et al., 2008]. Although, the elevation of ketone bodies may occur within a week of starting a VLCD, the complete process of keto-adaptation is measured in months, especially with regard to athletic performance [Volek, JS, et al., 2011b]. This study [Koeslag, JH, et al., 1980] evaluated the effect of training status, age, exercise duration and intensity, and dietary carbohydrate content on post-exercise ketosis. Of all the factors studied, dietary carbohydrate restriction was the critical factor in the development of post-exercise ketosis.

In those with T1D, dietary carbohydrate restriction requires reduced exogenous insulin doses, mimicking the normal reduction in insulin secretion, and results in a concomitant increase in glucagon secretion, both of which signal the fat cells to release fatty acids and the liver to make ketones from the fatty acids and to a lesser extent from ketogenic amino acids. The low insulin-to-glucagon ratio also signals the liver to break down glycogen to glucose (glycogenolysis) and to produce new glucose (gluconeogenesis) from pyruvate, lactate, glucogenic amino acids, glycerol, and acetone [Kaleta, C, et al., 2011]. There are two ketone bodies made by the liver, acetoacetic acid and β-hydroxybutyric acid. Both are weak acids that completely dissociate in the blood to form their conjugate bases (acetoacetate and β-hydroxybutyrate (BHB)) and a proton (H^+), i.e., acid. The acid is neutralized by bicarbonate (HCO_3^-) made by the kidneys, forming water (H_2O) and carbon dioxide (CO_2), and the CO_2 is excreted by the lungs. In nutritional ketosis, the blood pH and HCO_3^- are normal because the rate of ketone production is small relative to the kidney's and lung's ability to neutralize the acid. A third ketone, acetone, is formed by the spontaneous breakdown of acetoacetate in the blood. Some of the acetone is excreted by the lungs and gives the breath a fruity smell, most noticeable in those with DKA. Long-chain fatty acids are converted to ketones based on the body's need for ketones which is primarily determined by the degree of dietary carbohydrate restriction and the resulting insulin and glucagon levels. Interestingly, medium-chain fatty acids found in coconut, palm, and MCT oils are preferentially converted to ketones by the liver. BHB is the predominate ketone in the bloodstream and must be converted to acetoacetate in the mitochondria prior to being utilized to generate adenosine triphosphate (ATP): the universal cellular energy molecule. The predominance of BHB in the bloodstream reduces the amount of acetoacetate that breaks down to acetone and is lost in the breath. Both acetoacetate and BHB are excreted in the urine, but over time, the kidneys excrete fewer ketones resulting in lower urine ketone concentrations.

Ketones are a preferred fuel when glucose is less readily available for many key organs including the brain, heart, and skeletal muscle. The blood-brain barrier is not very permeable to fatty acids, so the brain, in particular, depends on ketones and glucose as a source of fuel. As the concentration of ketones in the blood increases, so does ketone utilization in the brain [Cunnane, SC, et al., 2016] while glucose utilization decreases proportionately [Zhang, Y, et al., 2013]. The ability to make ketones primarily from fat during periods of prolonged fasting (starvation ketosis) spares the breakdown of muscle protein that would otherwise be needed to make glucose via gluconeogenesis. This extends the survival of lean individuals without access to food from about two weeks to two months and is one of the reasons we have been able to survive as a species on earth for such a long time. Thus, ketosis rather than being an abnormal or dangerous state is actually a beneficial survival mechanism.

Measuring Ketones When Following a VLCD

While the ability to detect ketones in the urine has been available for many decades, in recent years, simple-to-use devices have been developed to measure ketones in the breath and blood. Urine ketone strips measure acetoacetate, breath ketone meters measure acetone, and blood ketone meters measure BHB. Measuring ketones is useful to those who choose to follow a VLCD to confirm that dietary carbohydrate restriction is sufficient enough to be in nutritional ketosis as well as for those with T1D to detect impending DKA or euDKA during an illness.

The least expensive of these methods is the urine ketone strip which measures the concentration of acetoacetate in the urine. Urine ketones ≥ 40 mg/dl (moderate) indicates nutritional ketosis. Although urine ketones remain positive indefinitely while in nutritional ketosis, urine ketones may become less positive a few months after beginning a VLCD because the kidneys do improve their ability to retain acetoacetate over time. Your state of hydration also influences the urine ketone strip results. Being mildly dehydrated will make urine ketones register higher, while being well-hydrated will make urine ketones register lower. Breath ketone meters are initially more expensive than urine strips or blood BHB meters/strips, but can be used thousands of times without buying any strips or supplies and are the least expensive method to measure ketones if you want to be able to measure them on a frequent basis. You simply exhale as much of the air in your lungs as you can into the device and you get a result. The third method is to measure BHB in the blood. When following a VLCD, nutritional ketosis is generally defined as having a blood BHB reading in the range 0.5–3.0 mM. Any BHB level > 0.5 mM indicates adequate carbohydrate restriction to achieve normal blood sugars. Higher levels of ketosis, in the range 3.1–6.0 mM, 1) can occur after exercise, 2) can occur when supplementing with coconut, palm, or medium-chain triglyceride (MCT) oil and/or exogenous ketones, 3) can occur with strict carbohydrate restriction (< 20 g/day), 4) may confer benefits beyond glycemic control, but definitive, long-term studies are lacking, and 5) are not dangerous. While I typically stay in the 0.5–2 mM BHB range, the highest blood BHB concentration I ever measured was 6.9 mM on Dec. 11, 2013 when I was trying elevate my BHB by supplementing with coconut oil at a dose of 4 tbsp/day. Personally, I have not noticed a correlation between ketone levels and exercise performance or blood glucose levels. Thus, the three reasons to check ketone levels are: 1) to confirm compliance with dietary carbohydrate restriction when one's intent is to follow a VLCD, 2) to understand your baseline ketone levels in the event of a future illness, and 3) to detect impending DKA or euDKA during an illness as indicated by ketone levels well above your baseline.

Diabetic Ketoacidosis

About 30–40% of children and 20% of adults present with DKA as the initial manifestation of T1D [Umpierrez, GE, et al., 2019]. DKA is caused by the uncontrolled production of ketones by the liver due to absolute or relative insulin deficiency. Absolute insulin deficiency occurs in those with undiagnosed T1D or when a person with T1D inappropriately reduces or stops taking exogenous insulin. Relative insulin deficiency occurs when insulin levels are inappropriately low and counterregulatory hormones are increased due to the stress of an illness. For example, when a person with T1D develops gastroenteritis and is unable to hold down food, they will need to reduce bolus and possibly basal insulin doses. However, DKA can result if they excessively reduce their insulin dosage in the setting of increased counterregulatory hormones. During DKA, low insulin and high counterregulatory hormone levels signal the liver to produce excessive quantities of glucose and ketones and reduces cellular glucose utilization. Because ketones are organic acids, when their rate of production exceeds the ability of the kidneys and lungs to excrete the excess acid, the blood becomes acidic with a pH < 7.3 and a serum HCO_3^- < 18 mEq/L resulting in a host of other metabolic problems [Kraut, JA, et al., 2010]. The hyperglycemia, combined with low insulin levels, result in a marked diuresis, increased urination, dehydration, and thirst. Of those who seek medical attention, only ≈ 1–5% will die from DKA [Nyenwe, EA, et al., 2016]. In the hospital, intravenous exogenous insulin and fluids quickly correct the insulin deficiency and dehydration, and stops the liver from making excess glucose and ketones allowing the hyperglycemia and acidosis to resolve. Of those who die in the hospital after presenting with DKA, most will die from the underlying illness that caused the DKA in the first place, most commonly a serious urinary tract infection, pneumonia, and/or sepsis, rather than from the metabolic disturbance of ketoacidosis itself [Umpierrez, GE, et al., 2019].

For those with T1D, it is advisable to own a blood ketone meter (Precision Xtra or Keto-Mojo) with BHB ketone strips on hand to be able to test for impending DKA in the event you become ill. If you choose to follow a VLCD, you should know your baseline ketone levels via periodic measurements. A significant increase in BHB concentration during an illness should prompt you to seek medical attention. If you choose not to periodically check ketone levels, this study [Sheikh-Ali, M, et al., 2008] found in the setting of an illness, presumably in those on a LFHCD, that a BHB reading ≥ 3 mM in children and ≥ 3.8 mM in adults was found to correlate with a diagnosis of DKA. Typically in DKA, blood glucose levels are in excess of 200 mg/dl (11.1 mM), but when following a LCD/VLCD, or in those taking an SGLT2 inhibitor (see Chapter 9), the blood glucose may be < 200 mg/dl (11.1 mM), i.e., euDKA. Thus, regardless of the blood glucose reading, a BHB significantly above your baseline, or a BHB ≥ 3 mM in children and ≥ 3.8 mM in adults, combined with feeling ill, should prompt you to seek medical attention.

Does nutritional ketosis from a VLCD increase one's risk of developing DKA? While no studies have been done to answer this question, my opinion is that 1) as long as a well-formulated VLCD is implemented, 2) blood sugars are monitored at least four times daily, 3) insulin is appropriately administered and adjusted to achieve normal or near-normal blood sugars, 4) and no illness or other known causes of DKA arise, then there should be no increased risk of developing DKA by being in nutritional ketosis.

Medium-Chain Triglycerides, Coconut Oil, and MCT Oil

Coconut oil pressed from coconut meat is a pure fat composed of medium- and long-chain fatty acids. Fatty acids vary in length from 3 to 24 carbons. Short-chain fatty acids are less than 8 carbons in length, medium-chain fatty acids range from 8 to 12 carbons in length, and long-chain fatty acids are more than 12 carbons in length. Coconut oil contains 49% lauric acid (12 carbons), 8% caprylic acid (10 carbons), and 7% capric acid (8 carbons). It turns out that medium-chain fatty acids and triglycerides are handled differently by the body than long-chain fatty acids and triglycerides. After absorption in the intestines, long-chain fatty acids and lauric acid are packaged into chylomicrons and carried in lymph vessels to the bloodstream, whereas, caprylic acid and capric acid are absorbed into the blood and carried directly to the liver. Think of chylomicrons as boats that transport long-chain fatty acids through the aqueous lymph and bloodstream to cells that need them for energy and to fat cells for storage. Medium-chain fatty acids are preferentially converted to ketones in the liver regardless of whether or not one is eating a LCD. By contrast, a smaller percentage of lauric acid is converted to ketones and its conversion is delayed by the transport time through the lymph vessels [McCarty, MF, et al., 2016]. Thus, lauric acid may prolong the elevation of blood ketone levels in conjunction with MCT oil. Lauric acid may also have potential benefits as an antimicrobial agent against pathogenic gut bacteria, e.g., clostridium difficile [Matsue, M, et al., 2019, Yang, H, et al., 2018]. Medium-chain triglyceride (MCT) oil is a refined form of coconut or palm oil containing about 75% caprylic acid and 25% capric acid, although there are other MCT oils with different proportions of caprylic acid and capric acid. Some MCT oils contain 100% caprylic acid which is even more readily converted to ketones than capric acid. I use both MCT and coconut oil as a source of energy and ketones in my keto chocolate mousse recipe even though they are refined, processed-food ingredients. MCT oil is also used in infant formulas, as part of a ketogenic VLCD for epilepsy, and for persons with abnormalities of fat absorption.

Known and Potential Benefits of Nutritional Ketosis

Research into the potential benefits of a ketogenic VLCD for many health conditions has grow in the past few decades and briefly includes the following:
1. Improvement in and reversal of T2D [Athinarayanan, SJ, et al., 2019].
2. Improvement in NAFLD [Browning, JD, et al., 2011].
3. Treatment of neurologic disorders including epilepsy, headache, neurotrauma, Alzheimer's disease, Parkinson's disease, sleep disorders, brain cancer, autism, chronic pain, and amyotrophic lateral sclerosis [de Mello, NP, et al., 2019, Gano, LB, et al., 2014, Kessler, SK, et al., 2011, Paoli, A, et al., 2013].
4. Reduction in free radial formation in mitochondria [Florence, TM, 1995, Veech, RL, et al., 2001] and improved mitochondrial function [Miller, VJ, et al., 2018].
5. Improved metabolic efficiency [Kashiwaya, Y, et al., 1994, Kashiwaya, Y, et al., 1997].
6. Ketones as a 'preferred fuel' compared to glucose [Owen, OE, et al., 1967, Zhang, Y, et al., 2013].
7. BHB inhibits histone deacetylases [Shimazu, T, et al., 2013].
8. BHB inhibits the NLRP3 inflammasome [Youm, Y, et al., 2015].
9. Reduces markers of chronic inflammation [Forsythe, CE, et al., 2008].
10. Modulation of mitophagy [Ludwig, DS, 2019].

11. Ketones as signaling agents [Newman, JC, et al., 2014a, Newman, JC, et al., 2014b, Newman, JC, et al., 2017].
12. Cardiovascular disease [Semenkovich, CF, 2006].
13. Cancer [Arcidiacono, B, et al., 2012, Goncalves, MD, et al., 2019].
14. Brain network stabilization by ketones [Mujica-Parodi, LR, et al., 2020]
15. Anti-catabolic effects of BHB [Koutnik, AP, et al., 2019].

For additional information on my blood ketone levels see my blog post #11 at https://ketogenicdiabeticathlete.wordpress.com/2015/12/12/11-ketone-metabolism-the-klchf-diet-bonus-topics/.

14 – Low-Carb Diet Myths

"How wonderful that we have met with a paradox.
Now we have some hope of making progress."
Niels Bohr, Awarded the Nobel Prize in Physics, 1922.

"In God we trust; all others must have data."
Bernard Fisher, MD, Breast cancer surgeon whose research ended the radical mastectomy.

Myth 1: A High-Protein LCD Can Injure Healthy Kidneys

As discussed in Chapter 4, dietary protein is an essential nutrient required to build and repair lean tissues like our organs, muscles, enzymes, and many hormones that regulate our body's chemistry. Our daily intake of dietary protein is determined by our body size and exercise regimen. The original paper that started the myth about dietary protein injuring healthy kidneys was published in 1982 [Brenner, BM, 1982]. Dr. Brenner made the argument that "modern ad libitum eating habits" was a likely candidate as a cause of continuing injury to kidneys in laboratory animals and humans with chronic kidney failure and **hypothesized** that this could also be responsible for the deterioration of renal (kidney) function as healthy individuals age. Dr. Brenner wrote, "Sustained rather than intermittent excesses of protein (and perhaps other solutes) in the diet impose similarly sustained increases in renal blood flow and glomerular filtration rates, which require that the 'reserve' glomeruli of the outer cortex be in use more or less continuously. Consequently, time-averaged pressures and flows in outer cortical glomeruli contribute to unrelenting 'intrarenal hypertension' and predispose even healthy people to progressive glomerular sclerosis and deterioration of renal function." First, Dr. Brenner acknowledged that his **hypothesis** was based on animal and human studies of chronic kidney failure, not in persons with normal kidney function. Second, he acknowledged that **'other solutes**,' other than dietary protein, could be responsible for the 'deterioration of renal function.' My point here is that while I agree that the modern diet of processed foods and the resulting insulin resistance and hyperinsulinemia is likely responsible for many chronic diseases including kidney disease 'as we age,' Dr. Brenner clearly was hypothesizing that dietary protein was potentially deleterious to healthy kidneys without sufficient evidence at the time. Since 1982, there has been no confirmation that dietary protein is, in fact, responsible for 'deterioration of renal function' in persons with normal kidney function. This review article [Martin, WF, et al., 2005] deals with this issue and concludes that, "While protein restriction may be appropriate for treatment of existing kidney disease, we find no significant evidence for a detrimental effect of high protein intakes on kidney function in healthy persons after centuries of a high protein Western diet." I also reviewed this topic in an article on the Diet Doctor website [Runyan, KR, 2019]. The guidelines provided in Table 4.11 regarding dietary protein intake are safe for those with healthy kidneys. Those with kidney disease should check with their nephrologist regarding a safe level of dietary protein intake.

Myth 2: A High-Protein VLCD is Not Ketogenic

As mentioned in Chapter 4, determining one's dietary protein needs is an inexact science and I suggested that if we must err, we do so on the side of 'more-than-enough.' The language of dietary protein intake and nutritional ketosis is confusing. You may read or hear phrases like, 'a high-protein VLCD is not ketogenic' or 'a LCHF diet must be moderate in protein and high in fat to be ketogenic.' However, there are no standardized definitions of 'low, moderate, or high' when it comes to protein, carbohydrate, and fat intake. The easiest way to know whether any particular diet is likely to be ketogenic or not is to simply calculate its ketogenic ratio (KR) using the Withrow equation, as discussed in Chapter 4. I have calculated the KR in Table 14.1 for a 70-kg person consuming either 2,000 kcal/day or 2,500 kcal/day using a wide range of dietary protein, carbohydrate, and fat intakes, in grams/day, consistent with a LCD/VLCD.

Table 14.1 — Ketogenic Ratio With Different Macronutrients

Protein (g/kg/d)	Protein (g/d)	Carbs (g/d)	Fat (g/d), 2,000 kcal/d	KR 2,000 kcal/d	Fat (g/d), 2,500 kcal/d	KR 2,500 kcal/d
1.0	70	20	182	2.49	238	2.92
1.5	105	20	167	2.03	222	2.41
2.3	161	20	142	1.58	197	1.89
1.0	70	30	178	2.17	233	2.58
1.5	105	30	162	1.81	218	2.17
2.3	161	30	137	1.44	193	1.74
1.0	70	40	173	1.92	229	2.30
1.5	105	40	158	1.63	213	1.97
2.3	161	40	133	1.32	188	1.60
1.0	70	50	169	1.71	224	2.07
1.5	105	50	153	1.48	209	1.79

Master Type 1 Diabetes

2.3	161	50	128	1.21	184	1.48
1.0	70	60	164	1.54	220	1.88
1.5	105	60	149	1.34	204	1.64
2.3	161	60	124	1.12	180	1.38

As shown in Table 14.1, a 30 g/day dietary carbohydrate intake results in a KR ≥ 1.7 [Zilberter T, et al., 2018], for all dietary protein intakes at 2,500 kcal/day, but not at 2.3 g/kg/d dietary protein intake and 2,000 kcal/day. Examination of Table 14.1 reveals that the apparent antiketogenic effect of increasing dietary protein intake from 1.0 to 2.3 g/kg/d is magnified by the corresponding reduction in dietary fat (which is 90% ketogenic) which is required to keep caloric intake constant. Even so, at a 30 g/day dietary carbohydrate intake, a 130% increase in dietary protein intake from 1.0 to 2.3 g/kg BW/day results in only a 33% decrease in the KR, from 2.58 to 1.74, at 2,500 kcal/day. As pointed out in Chapter 4, the potential for a diet to result in nutritional ketosis according to the Withrow equation, $KR = (0.9\ F + 0.46\ P) \div (C + 0.58\ P + 0.1\ F)$, is determined primarily by its dietary carbohydrate and fat content and less so by its dietary protein content. Dietary protein is mildly antiketogenic because it is mildly insulinogenic, dietary carbohydrate is very antiketogenic because it is very insulinogenic, and dietary fat is minimally antiketogenic because it is minimally insulinogenic. Insulin inhibits liver mitochondrial ketone synthesis by multiple mechanisms [Grabacka, M, et al., 2016] including inhibition of the rate-limiting enzyme in ketone synthesis, HMG-CoA synthase. Personally, I have been in nutritional ketosis since beginning my VLCD in 2012 while my dietary carbohydrate has ranged from 30–70 grams/day, dietary protein from 1.8–2.3 g/kg/day, with enough dietary fat to maintain my desired bodyweight and support my athletic pursuits. My higher than average daily caloric intake, 35–40 kcal/kg/day, allows for more dietary fat intake which increases the KR of my diet and can compensate for a higher dietary carbohydrate and/or protein intake. In summary, both a high-protein VLCD and a moderate-protein LCHF diet may or may not be ketogenic depending on the dietary carbohydrate and fat intake, but you can choose whether or not you want to be in nutritional ketosis by using the Withrow equation to design your dietary macronutrient profile and then confirm whether or not you are in nutritional ketosis by measuring your ketones via urine, breath, or blood.

There also seems to be some confusion regarding the metabolic fate of any 'excess' dietary protein we might be consuming. Some believe that all or a large portion of 'excess' dietary protein is converted to glucose and that this, in turn, might increase insulin requirements, lead to hyperglycemia, or inhibit nutritional ketosis. First, it is difficult to know whether or not we are consuming an excess of dietary protein. Second, while production of glucose in the liver via gluconeogenesis is one potential metabolic fate of the glucogenic amino acids, dietary protein can also be converted to acetyl-CoA to make ATP in the mitochondria as an energy source or be converted to fatty acids for use throughout the body or stored in fat cells, and in the case of ketogenic amino acids, be converted to ketones for use throughout the body. In humans, up to 10% of energy needs are met from protein catabolism and 90% from dietary carbohydrates and fat [Garrett, RH, et al., 2013]. Excess dietary protein is thus converted to glucose via gluconeogenesis only to the extent that the body needs glucose. Gluconeogenesis is driven by demand for glucose, not supply of 'excess' amino acids. This study [Fromentin, C, et al., 2013] used multiple stable isotopes to measure endogenous glucose production (EGP) by the liver from dietary protein (eggs) in eight healthy subjects consuming 1.4 grams protein/kg/day for 5 days. "During the 8 hours after egg ingestion [containing 23 g protein], 50.4 g of glucose was produced, but only 3.9 g originated from dietary amino acids (AA). Our results show that the total postprandial contribution of dietary AA to EGP was small in humans habituated to a diet medium-rich in proteins, even after an overnight fast and in the absence of carbohydrates from the meal." Third, 'excess' dietary protein will slightly increase insulin requirements, but if insulin is dosed properly, will not cause hyperglycemia. For those choosing to be in nutritional ketosis by following a VLCD, limiting dietary protein for fear than any excess will be converted to glucose should not be a concern since dietary protein is only mildly antiketogenic.

In summary, the majority of calories in both LCD and VLCD comes from dietary fat, so technically, they are both 'high-fat.' Dietary protein should not be moderated or restricted, in my opinion, due to the numerous benefits on satiety and preservation of lean muscle and bone mass especially in older individuals (age ≥ 74 years) due to anabolic resistance [Wall, BT, et al., 2015]. The presence and degree of nutritional ketosis is primarily determined by the degree of dietary carbohydrate restriction and the 'high-fat' nature of a VLCD with a minor influence from its dietary protein content. Each individual can choose whether or not they want to be in nutritional ketosis and use the Withrow equation as a guide to formulate the macronutrients in their LCD/VLCD.

Myth 3: Dietary Carbohydrates Are Needed For Brain Energy

Various 'authoritative sources' may state that you must consume at least 130 grams of dietary carbohydrate each day to meet the brain's requirement for glucose. If this were literally true, no one would be able to go without food for more than one day which we know is not the case. The reference often cited is the Institute of Medicine's *Dietary Reference*

Intakes for Energy, Carbohydrate, Fiber, Fat, Fatty acids, Cholesterol, Protein, and Amino Acids [Institute of Medicine, 2005]. It is true that this report does state, "The Recommended Dietary Allowance for carbohydrate is set at 130 g/d for adults and children (Table S-2)." Their justification for this requirement is that, "This amount of glucose should be sufficient to supply the brain with fuel in the absence of a rise in circulating acetoacetate and β-hydroxybutyrate (BHB) concentrations greater than that observed in an individual after an overnight fast." However, they do not provide a reason why acetoacetate and BHB concentrations should not rise above the levels observed after an overnight fast. On page 289 in this report, it is stated that, "Nevertheless, it should be recognized that the brain can still receive enough glucose from the metabolism of the glycerol component of fat and from the gluconeogenic amino acids in protein when a very low carbohydrate diet is consumed." On page 275, they write, "The lower limit of dietary carbohydrate compatible with life apparently is zero, provided that adequate amounts of protein and fat are consumed." And on page 361, they state, "Dietary and functional fibers are not essential nutrients, so inadequate intakes do not result in biochemical or clinical symptoms of a deficiency." While not an essential nutrient, it is possible that dietary fiber is beneficial to persons with diabetes [Zhang, T, et al., 2018]. Humans do not have the enzymes needed to break the chemical bonds between the glucose molecules in dietary fiber, but the bacteria in our gut microbiome do have such enzymes. These bacteria are able to utilize dietary fiber to produce short-chain fatty acids which are used as a source of energy for our intestinal cells [Morrison, DJ, et al., 2016].

Myth 4: Low-Carbohydrate Diets Are Nutrient Deficient

It is possible to design any diet, including a LCD/VLCD, to be nutrient deficient if that is one's intent. As discussed in Chapter 4, it is fairly straightforward to design a nutrient-dense LCD that meets 100% of the RDA for vitamins and minerals using <u>cronometer.com</u>. I suspect that those making a claim that a LCD is nutrient deficient haven't taken the time to design a nutrient-sufficient LCD. Since the RDA for micronutrients is not bodyweight-based, it is possible that a short-statured female seeking to lose body fat might not be consuming enough food to be able to meet 100% of the RDA for some micronutrients and may need to take a vitamin and mineral supplement while losing weight. I take several supplements including magnesium chloride, potassium chloride (Morton's Lite Salt), vitamin B12 0.5 mg 2x/week, vitamin D 5,000 IU 3x/week, and vitamin C 200 mg daily just to be sure I get enough.

Myth 5: Low-Carbohydrate Diets Cause Osteoporosis

Osteoporosis occurs when the rate of bone loss exceeds the rate of bone regeneration and occurs most commonly in small-framed, white and asian, women as they age. Risk factors for osteoporosis include lack of dietary protein, calcium, and vitamin D intake, drinking alcohol, smoking, and lack of weight-bearing and resistance exercise. The myth about loss of bone calcium on a high-protein LCD stems from the observation that increasing dietary protein intake increases urinary calcium excretion and generates acid as part of its normal metabolism. "One estimate is that there is a 50% increase in urinary calcium associated with doubling protein intake or roughly 1 mg urinary calcium for every gram of dietary protein. However, the increase in urinary calcium observed with purified proteins or amino acid infusions is not readily observed with food sources of protein" [Heaney, RP, 2006]. "Urinary calcium has been found to be increased with acid-forming foods, such as meat, fish, eggs, and cereal, and negatively associated with plant foods and is likely determined by the acid-base status of the total diet. The kidneys excrete the acid generated from the normal degradation of proteins, but requires sufficient dietary potassium intake to maintain electroneutrality. Thus, insufficient potassium in the diet can reduce net acid excretion." This relationship may explain the reported beneficial influence of fruit and vegetables, the major dietary source of potassium, on bone health" [Heaney, RP, et al., 2008]. "In addition to calcium in the presence of an adequate supply of vitamin D, dietary proteins represent key nutrients for bone health and thereby function in the prevention of osteoporosis" [Bonjour, JP, 2011]. This 2-year weight-loss study [Foster, GD, et al., 2010] measured bone mineral density using DEXA at baseline and at 6, 12, and 24 months and found no differences in bone mineral density between the two diet groups: a 20-gram/day VLCD compared to a calorie-restricted LFHCD group over 2 years. A similar weight-loss study [Brinkworth, GD, et al., 2016] also found no difference in bone mineral density between two calorie-restricted diet groups: a 20-gram/day VLCD (4% of total energy as carbohydrate, 35% protein, and 61% fat) group compared to a LFHCD (46% of total energy as carbohydrate, 24% protein and 30% fat) group over 1 year. Other controlled diet studies have also been unable to detect any worsening of bone mineral density or markers of bone cell turnover when following a VLCD [Carter, JD, et al., 2006, Hu, T, et al., 2016].

Myth 6: Low-Carbohydrate Diets Cause Muscle Wasting

A number of studies have examined changes in lean muscle mass with a LCD/VLCD, some in normal weight individuals, some in combination with an exercise training program, and some in overweight or obese individuals undergoing weight loss. This small 6-week clinical trial [Volek, JS, et al., 2002] examined changes in fat mass and fat-free mass in twelve normal-weight men who agreed to adopt a calorie-unrestricted VLCD (8% energy from carbohydrate) compared to eight normal-weight men (controls) who continued their habitual diet (58% energy from carbohydrate). The study found that the VLCD resulted in a significant reduction in fat mass (−24.6% vs. 0.0%) and a concomitant increase in fat-free mass (+1.8% vs. +0.6%) that may have been, in part, mediated by the reduction in circulating insulin concentrations. This study [Paoli, A, et al., 2012] measured both strength and body composition in eight elite artistic gymnasts before and after a 30-day VLCD and compared it to the athletes' usual Western diet. The VLCD resulted in significant improvements in bodyweight (from 69.6 kg to 68.0 kg), fat mass (from 5.3 kg to 3.4 kg), and non-significant increase in muscle mass (from 37.6 to 37.9 kg) compared to the Western diet. The authors concluded that the preservation of muscle mass and strength and the loss of fat mass with the VLCD might be particularly advantageous for athletes who compete in sports with bodyweight divisions. In this study [Gregory, RM, et al., 2017], the authors found that a VLCD (< 50 grams carbohydrate/day) combined with six weeks of CrossFit training lead to significant decreases in percent body fat (−2.60% vs. −0.01%) and fat mass (−2.83 kg vs. −0.06 kg) with no significant difference in fat-free mass or athletic performance compared to the control group following their usual diet. This commentary article [Manninen, AH, et al., 2006] reviewed a number of weight-loss studies and concluded that "... it appears, from most literature studied, that a VLCD is, if anything, protective against muscle protein catabolism during energy restriction, provided that it contains adequate amounts of protein."

Myth 7: Low-Carbohydrate Whole Foods Are Expensive

Some have the perception that convenient processed foods including fast foods, ready-to-eat foods, and restaurant foods are less expensive than healthful low-carb foods from the grocery store. I have been told by some patients that they can't afford to buy healthful foods, I believe, as an excuse to continue their current eating habits. Just in case you have that same excuse in mind, this section is for you. Logic tells you that the food industry knows people are willing to pay more money for their convenience. They are appealing to a natural trait of humans to expend the least effort to get the most calories. This trait worked well and helped us survive as a species for hundreds of thousands of years when we hunted and gathered our food. But in our current food environment, this trait works against us. Thus to transform our health in a positive direction, we need to eat real whole foods from a grocery store, farmer's market, or out of our own, or community, garden and cook that food at home. Having done it myself since 2012, I can tell you eating whole low-carb food is far less expensive.

The single most economical and healthful low-carb food is eggs. The next most economical source of protein and fat is chicken, followed by beef, pork, and fish. Buying food in larger quantities at a lower cost per pound and freezing it raw or pre-cooked saves money. For busy people working and going to school, a week's worth of food can be cooked and portioned out in containers on the weekend and refrigerated or frozen for the next week. By preparing food this way, I have no doubt it is less expensive than buying any prepared, processed food. And even if healthful foods were more expensive, the reduction in medical costs due to smaller insulin doses, fewer physician visits, and fewer hospitalizations would more than make up for any increase in the cost of healthful low-carb foods.

Myth 8: Glargine (Lantus) Insulin Increases Cancer Risk

Even though this myth is not related to the LCD, I wanted to cover this topic since I have been asked numerous times on my blog at https://ketogenicdiabeticathlete.wordpress.com about 'glargine (Lantus) being associated with an increased risk of cancer.' The original study [Hemkens, LG, et al., 2009] that started this myth about glargine (Lantus) and cancer risk was an epidemiological study initiated by the "largest German statutory health insurance fund" based on reimbursement considerations. First, this study's applicability to those with T1D is doubtful since the authors state: "No definite distinction between diabetes types 1 and 2 could be made on the basis of these data." The authors state that the study found "a slightly lower cancer incidence in the glargine group." Yes, you read that correctly. Then they used an unconventional and fundamentally flawed analysis that adjusted for the lower glargine dosages to conclude the opposite of what was actually found: "the cancer incidence with glargine was higher than expected compared with human insulin," an unsupportable conclusion from the data [Owens, DR, 2012]. They also admit that "we cannot entirely exclude the possibility that some known or unknown factors could have influenced both the dose of human insulin and insulin analogues and the risk of cancer, especially given that the groups being compared were clinically dissimilar. Ultimately, only a randomised controlled trial could dispel these concerns." The authors add "The findings underline the necessity for a prospective, randomised, controlled, long-term study that is designed and sufficiently powered to evaluate insulin analogues with regard to their effects on morbidity and mortality in patients with diabetes."

Other studies were unable to find an excess cancer risk including a 5-year RCT comparing NPH and glargine [Rosenstock, J, et al., 2009] or when the combined RCT experience of malignancies in 31 studies, 12 in type 1 diabetes and 19 in type 2 diabetes, using glargine were evaluated [Home, PD, et al., 2009]. Finally, the *Consensus Report on Cancer and Diabetes* by the American Diabetes Association and American Cancer Society concluded that "further research is needed to clarify these issues and evaluate if insulin glargine is more strongly associated with cancer risk compared with other insulins" [Giovannucci, E, et al., 2010]. "The chapter on whether insulin glargine per se is an independent risk factor for cancer should now be closed" [Owens, DR, 2012].

Diabetes And Weight-Management Coaching

If you would like some assistance with managing blood sugars, bodyweight, or other aspects of T1D, I can help you via my coaching service. Since I work exclusively online, I can't do a physical examination and I don't have access to your medical records, so I can't give medical advice. I can help you better manage your blood sugars in conjunction with your physician at https://ketogenicdiabeticathlete.wordpress.com/coaching/.

Comments, Book Reviews, Suggestions, Are All Welcome

While I understand that their are as many ways to treat T1D as there are those who have it, I have presented in this book, a simple, low-tech, low-cost method to normalize blood sugars. My method is not the only way to achieve normal blood sugars. Others may choose a different dietary approach, want to live a more flexible or unregimented lifestyle, or use an insulin pump, CGM, or artificial pancreas to accomplish their goals, which is great if they can accomplish their goals. I sincerely hope that those who read this book and apply the strategies within, will feel better for having done so, improve their blood sugars, and prevent, or improve, long-term diabetic complications. If you feel this book has helped you, I would appreciate it if you could write a positive review of the book on Amazon so that others can benefit from your experience with it. If you have suggestions for improvement or would like to share your experience utilizing the strategies in this book, I would appreciate hearing from you at: krunyanmd@gmail.com.

Table of Abbreviations

Abbreviation	Item
ADA	American Diabetes Association
ALA	Alpha-linolenic acid
ApoA-1	Apolipoprotein A-1
ApoB	Apolipoprotein B
BHB	β-hydroxybutyrate
BID	Bolus insulin dose(s)
CGM	Continuous glucose monitor(s)
COV	Coefficient of Variation
CVD	Cardiovascular disease
DCCT	Diabetes Control and Complications Trial
DEXA	Dual energy x-ray absorptiometry
DHA	Docosahexaenoic acid
EFSA	The European Food Safety Authority
EPA	Eicosapentaenoic acid
HDL-C	High-density lipoprotein cholesterol
hsCRP	High-sensitivity C reactive protein
IG	Interstitial glucose
IL-1β	Interleukin-1β
IL-6	Interleukin-6
IU	International unit, measure of insulin dose

KR	Ketogenic ratio
LA	linoleic acid
LCD	Low-carbohydrate diet (51–100 grams/day)
LCT	Long-chain triglyceride
LDL-C	Low-density lipoprotein cholesterol
LDL-P	Low-density lipoprotein particle number
LFHCD	Low-fat high-carbohydrate diet
Lp(a)	Lipoprotein a
LTB4	Leukotriene B4
MCT	Medium-chain triglyceride
mM	Millimoles per liter, mmol/l, mmol/L
MUFA	Monounsaturated fatty acids
NAFLD	Non-alcoholic fatty liver disease
NPH insulin	Neutral Protamine Hagedorn insulin
PAI-1	Plasminogen activator inhibitor-1
PGE2	Prostaglandin E_2
PUFA	Polyunsaturated fatty acids
RCT	Randomized controlled trial
RDA	Recommended daily allowance, USDA
RDI	Recommended daily intake, USDA
ROS	Reactive oxygen species
SDBG	Standard deviation of blood glucose
SDIG	Standard deviation of interstitial glucose

sdLDL	Small-dense low-density lipoprotein
SFA	Saturated fatty acids
SMBG	Self-monitored blood glucose
T1D	Type 1 diabetes mellitus
T2D	Type 2 diabetes mellitus
TC	Total cholesterol
TDID	Total daily insulin dose
TG	Serum triglycerides
TNFα	Tumor necrosis factor alpha
TXA2	Thromboxane A2
VLCD	Very low-carbohydrate diet (20–50 grams/day)
VLDL	Very low-density lipoprotein
VLDL-C	Very low-density lipoprotein cholesterol

Table of References

2018 Physical Activity Guidelines Advisory Committee, 2nd edition, 2018. *2018 Physical Activity Guidelines Advisory Committee Scientific Report*, Washington, DC, U.S. Department of Health and Human Services, 2018.

Achenbach, P, et al., 2005. Natural History of Type 1 Diabetes, *Diabetes*, 54 (Suppl. 2): S25–S31.

Ahrens, EH, et al., 1961. Carbohydrate-induced and fat-induced lipemia, *Trans Ass Amer Physicians*, 74: 134.

Al Jobori, H, et al., 2017. Determinants of the Increase in Fasting Plasma Ketone Concentration during SGLT2 Inhibition in NGT, IFG and T2D Patients, *Diabetes Obes Metab*, 19(6): 809–13.

Albrink, MJ, et al., 1959. Serum Triglycerides in Coronary Artery Disease, *AMA Arch Intern Med*, 103(1): 4–8.

Albrink, MJ, et al., 1961. Serum Lipids, Hypertension, and Coronary Artery Disease, *Am J Med*, (31)1: 4–23.

Ames, BN, 2006. Low micronutrient intake may accelerate the degenerative diseases of aging through allocation of scarce micronutrients by triage, *PNAS*, 103(47): 17589–94.

Antonio, J, et al., 2014. The effects of consuming a high protein diet (4.4 g/kg/d) on body composition in resistance-trained individuals, *J Int Soc Sports Nutr*, 11: 19.

Antonio, J, et al., 2018. Case Reports on Well-Trained Bodybuilders: Two Years on a High Protein Diet, *J Exer Physiol*, 21(1): 14–24.

Araujo, J, et al., 2018. Prevalence of Optimal Metabolic Health in American Adults: National Health and Nutrition Examination Survey 2009–2016, *Metab Syndr Relat Disord*, 20(20): 1–7.

Arcidiacono, B, et al., 2012. Insulin Resistance and Cancer Risk: An Overview of the Pathogenetic Mechanisms, *Exp Diabetes Res*, Article ID 789174.

Aronson, D, et al., 2002. How hyperglycemia promotes atherosclerosis: molecular mechanisms, *Cardiovasc Diabetol*, 1: 1.

Athinarayanan, SJ, et al., 2019. Long-Term Effects of a Novel Continuous Remote Care Intervention Including Nutritional Ketosis for the Management of Type 2 Diabetes: A 2-Year Non-randomized Clinical Trial, *Front Endocrinol*, 10: 348.

Austin, MA, et al., 1988. Low-Density Lipoprotein Subclass Patterns and Risk of Myocardial Infarction, *JAMA*, 260: 1917–21.

Bailey, TS, 2017. Clinical Implications of Accuracy Measurements of Continuous Glucose Sensors, *Diabetes Technol Ther*, 19: 2, S51–S54.

Bally, L, et al., 2016. Accuracy of Continuous Glucose Monitoring During Differing Exercise Conditions, *Diabetes Res Clin Pract*, 112: 1–5.

Bao, J, et al., 2009. Food insulin index: physiologic basis for predicting insulin demand evoked by composite meals, *J Clin Nutr*, 90: 986–92.

Beck, JK, et al., 2015. Outpatient Management of Pediatric Type 1 Diabetes, *J Pediatr Pharmacol Ther*, 20(5): 344–57.

Beck, RW, et al., 2010. Variation of interstitial glucose measurements assessed by continuous glucose monitors in healthy, nondiabetic individuals, *Diabetes Care*, 33(6): 1297–99.

Bekiari, E, et al., 2018. Artificial pancreas treatment for outpatients with type 1 diabetes: systematic review and meta-analysis, *BMJ*, 361: k1310.

Bergen, G, et al., 2016. Falls and Fall Injuries Among Adults Aged ≥65 Years — United States, 2014, *Morb Mortal Wkly Rep*, 65(37): 993–8.

Bergeron, N, et al., 2019. Effects of Red Meat, White Meat, and Nonmeat Protein Sources on Atherogenic Lipoprotein Measures in the Context of Low Compared With High Saturated Fat Intake: A Randomized Controlled Trial, *Am J Clin Nutr*, 110(1): 24–33.

Bernstein, RK, 2011. *Dr. Bernstein's Diabetes Solution: The Complete Guide To Achieving Normal Blood Sugars*, 4th edition, Little, Brown and Company.

Biagi, L, et al., 2018. Accuracy of Continuous Glucose Monitoring before, during, and after Aerobic and Anaerobic Exercise in Patients with Type 1 Diabetes Mellitus, *Biosensors*, 2018, 8(22): 1–8.

Bird, SR, 2017. Update on the effects of physical activity on insulin sensitivity in humans, *BMJ Open Sport Exerc Med*, 2: e000143.

Bohé, J, et al., 2001. Latency and duration of stimulation of human muscle protein synthesis during continuous infusion of amino acids, *J Physiol*, 532(2): 575–9.

Bonjour, JP, 2011. Protein intake and bone health, *Int J Vitam Nutr Res*, 81(2–3), 134–42.

Borghouts, LB, et al., 1999. Exercise and Insulin Sensitivity: A Review, *Int J Sports Med*, 20: 1–12.

Braffett, BH, et al., 2019a. Association of Insulin Dose, Cardiometabolic Risk Factors, and Cardiovascular Disease in Type 1 Diabetes During 30 Years of Follow-up in the DCCT/EDIC Study, *Diabetes Care*, 42(4): 657–64.

Braffett, BH, et al., 2019b. Mediation of the association of smoking and microvascular complications by glycemic control in type 1 diabetes, *PLoS ONE*, 14(1): e0210367.

Brenner, BM, 1982. Dietary Protein Intake and the Progressive Nature of Kidney Disease: The Role of Hemodynamically Mediated Glomerular Injury in the Pathogenesis of Progressive Glomerular Sclerosis in Aging, Renal Ablation, and Intrinsic Renal Disease, *N Engl J Med*, 307: 652–659.

Brinkworth, GD, et al., 2016. Long-term effects of a very low carbohydrate weight loss diet and an isocaloric low-fat diet on bone health in obese adults, *Nutrition*, 32(9), 1033–36.

Brown, SA, et al., 2019. Six-Month Randomized, Multicenter Trial of Closed-Loop Control in Type 1 Diabetes, *N Engl J Med*, 381: 1707–17.

Browning, JD, et al., 2011. Short-term weight loss and hepatic triglyceride reduction: evidence of a metabolic advantage with dietary carbohydrate restriction, *Am J Clin Nutr*, 93: 1048–52.

Brownlee, M, et al., 2006. Glycemic Variability: A Hemoglobin A1c–Independent Risk Factor for Diabetic Complications, *JAMA*, 295(14): 1707–8.

Cahill, GF, 1983. President's Address: Starvation, *Trans Am Clin Climatol Assoc*, 94: 1–21.

Cahill, GF, et al., 2003. Ketoacids? Good Medicine?, *Trans Am Clin Climatol Assoc*, 114: 149–63.

Carter, JD, et al., 2006. The effect of a low-carbohydrate diet on bone turnover, *Osteoporos Int*, 17(9): 1398–403.

Chaston, TB, et al., 2007. Changes in fat-free mass during significant weight loss: a systematic review, *Int J Obes*, 31: 743–50.

Chaturvedi, N, et al., 1995. The Relationship Between Smoking and Microvascular Complications in the EURODIAB IDDM Complications Study, *Diabetes Care*, 18(6): 785–92.

Chia, JSJ, et al., 2017. A1 beta-casein milk protein and other environmental predisposing factors for type 1 diabetes, *Nutr Diabetes*, 7, e274.

Chimen, M, et al., 2012. What are the health benefits of physical activity in type 1 diabetes mellitus? A literature review, Diabetologia, 55(3): 542–51.

Cicero, AFG, et al., 2015. Middle and Long-Term Impact of a Very Low-Carbohydrate Ketogenic Diet on Cardiometabolic Factors: A Multi-Center, Cross-Sectional, Clinical Study, *High Blood Press Cardiovasc Prev*, 22: 389–94.

Cipryan, L, et al., 2018. Effects of a 4-Week Very Low-Carbohydrate Diet on High-Intensity Interval Training Responses, *J Sci Med Sport*, 17: 259–68.

Clarke, SF, et al., 2012. A history of blood glucose meters and their role in self-monitoring of diabetes mellitus, *British J Biomed Sci*, 69(2).

Colberg, SR, et al., 2013. Blood Glucose Responses to Type, Intensity, Duration, and Timing of Exercise, *Diabetes Care*, 36: e177.

Colberg, SR, et al., 2015. Physical Activity and Type 1 Diabetes: Time for a Rewire?, *J Diabetes Sci Technol*, 9(3): 609–18.

Colquitt, J, et al., 2003. Are analogue insulins better than soluble in continuous subcutaneous insulin infusion? Results of a meta-analysis, *Diabet Med*, 20: 863–6.

Cordain, L, 2011. *The Paleo Diet*, John Wiley & Sons, Inc.

Cortés, ME, et al., 2014. The effects of hormonal contraceptives on glycemic regulation, *Linacre Q*, 81(3): 209–18.

Crofts, CAP, et al., 2015. Hyperinsulinemia: A unifying theory of chronic disease?, *Diabesity*, 1(4): 34–43.

Cryer, PE, 2012. *Hypoglycemia In Diabetes: Pathophysiology, Prevalence, and Prevention*, 2nd edition, American Diabetes Association.

Cunnane, SC, et al., 2016. Can Ketones Help Rescue Brain Fuel Supply in Later Life? Implications for Cognitive Health during Aging and the Treatment of Alzheimer's Disease, *Front Mol Neurosci*, 9: 53.

Dandona, P, et al., 2005. Metabolic Syndrome: A Comprehensive Perspective Based on Interactions Between Obesity, Diabetes, and Inflammation, *Circulation*, 111: 1448–54.

Danese, E, et al., 2015. Advantages and Pitfalls of Fructosamine and Glycated Albumin in the Diagnosis and Treatment of Diabetes, *J Diabetes Sci Technol*, 9(2): 169–76.

Danne, T, et al., 2019. International Consensus on Risk Management of Diabetic Ketoacidosis in Patients With Type 1 Diabetes Treated With Sodium–Glucose Cotransporter (SGLT) Inhibitors, *Diabetes Care*, 42: 1147–54.

de Cabo, R, et al., 2019. Effects of Intermittent Fasting on Health, Aging, and Disease, *N Engl J Med*, 381: 2541–51.

de Ferranti, SD, et al., 2014. Type 1 Diabetes Mellitus and Cardiovascular Disease: A Scientific Statement From the American Heart Association and American Diabetes Association, *Diabetes Care*, 37: 2843–63.

de Mello, NP, et al., 2019. Insulin and Autophagy in Neurodegeneration, *Front Neurosci*, 13: 491.

Deichmann, R, et al., 2010. Coenzyme Q10 and Statin-Induced Mitochondrial Dysfunction, *Ochsner J*, 10(1): 16–21.

DiFeliceantonio, AG, et al., 2018. Supra-Additive Effects of Combining Fat and Carbohydrate on Food Reward, *Cell Metab*, 28: 33–44.

Dijkstra, A, et al., 2017. Whole Blood Donation Affects the Interpretation of Hemoglobin A1c, *PLoS ONE*, 12(1): e0170802.

Dimitriadis, G, et al., 2011. Insulin effects in muscle and adipose tissue, *Diabetes Res Clin Pract*, 93S: S52–9.

DiNicolantonio, JJ, et al., 2018. Omega-6 vegetable/seed oils as a driver of coronary heart disease: the oxidized linoleic acid hypothesis, *Open Heart*, 5: 1–6.

Divers, J, et al., 2020. Trends in Incidence of Type 1 and Type 2 Diabetes Among Youths — Selected Counties and Indian Reservations, United States, 2002–2015, *MMWR*, (69)6: 161–165.

Donga, E, et al., 2010. A single night of partial sleep deprivation induces insulin resistance in multiple metabolic pathways in healthy subjects, *J Clin Endocrinol Metab*, 95: 2963–8.

Ekhlaspour, L, et al., 2017. Comparative Accuracy of 17 Point-of- Care Glucose Meters, *J Diabetes Sci Technol*, 11(3): 558–66.

Emanuele, NV, et al., 1998. Consequences of Alcohol Use in Diabetics, *Alcohol Health Res World*, 22(3): 211–9.

Fanelli, CG, et al., 1993. Meticulous Prevention of Hypoglycemia Normalizes the Glycemic Thresholds and Magnitude of Most of Neuroendocrine Responses to, Symptoms of, and Cognitive Function During Hypoglycemia in Intensively Treated Patients With Short-Term IDDM, *Diabetes*, 42: 1683–89.

Farquhar, JW, et al., 1966. Glucose, Insulin, and Triglyceride Responses to High and Low Carbohydrate Diets in Man, *J Clin Invest*, 45(1): 1648–56.

Fasano, A, 2011. Zonulin and Its Regulation of Intestinal Barrier Function: The Biological Door to Inflammation, Autoimmunity, and Cancer, *Physiol Rev*, 91: 151–75.

Feinman, RD, 2006. Low carbohydrate diets improve atherogenic dyslipidemia even in the absence of weight loss, *Nutr Metab*, 3: 24.

Feinman, RD, et al., 2015. Dietary carbohydrate restriction as the first approach in diabetes management: Critical review and evidence base, *Nutrition*, 31: 1–13.

Fenech, MF, 2010. Dietary reference values of individual micronutrients and nutriomes for genome damage prevention: current status and a road map to the future, *Am J Clin Nutr*, 91 (suppl): 1438S–54S.

Ferreira-Hermosillo, A, et al., 2014. Utility of the waist-to-height ratio, waist circumference and body mass index in the screening of metabolic syndrome in adult patients with type 1 diabetes mellitus, *Diabetol Metab Syndr*, 6(32): 1–7.

Filippi, CM, et al., 2008. Viral trigger for type 1 diabetes: pros and cons, *Diabetes*, 57.

Florence, TM, 1995. The role of free radicals in disease, *Aust New Zeal J Ophthalmol*, 23(1).

Forsythe, CE, et al., 2008. Comparison of Low Fat and Low Carbohydrate Diets on Circulating Fatty Acid Composition and Markers of Inflammation, *Lipids*, 43: 65–77.

Foster, GD, et al., 2010. Weight and Metabolic Outcomes After 2 Years on a Low-Carbohydrate Versus Low-Fat Diet: A Randomized Trial, *Ann Intern Med*, 153(3), 147–57.

Foster, NC, et al., 2019. State of Type 1 Diabetes Management and Outcomes from the T1D Exchange in 2016–2018, *Diabetes Technol Ther*, 21(2).

Freckmann, G, et al., 2007. Continuous Glucose Profiles in Healthy Subjects under Everyday Life Conditions and after Different Meals, *J Diabetes Sci Technol*, 1(5): 695–703.

Fromentin, C, et al., 2013. Dietary Proteins Contribute Little to Glucose Production, Even Under Optimal Gluconeogenic Conditions in Healthy Humans, *Diabetes*, 62: 1435–42.

Frontoni, S, et al., 2013. Glucose variability: An emerging target for the treatment of diabetes mellitus, *Diabetes Res Clin Pract*, 102(2): 86–95.

Fuchsjäger-Mayrl, G, et al., 2002. Exercise training improves vascular endothelial function in patients with type 1 diabetes, Diabetes Care, 25(10): 1795–801.

Ganiats, T, 2006. Variability in Insulin Action: Mechanisms, Implications, and Recent Advances, *Internet J Fam Pract*, 5(2).

Gano, LB, et al., 2014. Ketogenic diets, mitochondria, and neurological diseases, *J Lipid Res*, 55: 2211–28.

Garrett, RH, et al., 2013. *Biochemistry, 5th edition, International Edition*, Brooks/Cole, Cengage Learning, pages 878–86.

Garthe, I, et al., 2011. Effect of two different weight-loss rates on body composition and strength and power-related performance in elite athletes, *Int J Sport Nutr Exerc Metab*, 21: 97–104.

Gibson, AA, et al., 2015. Do ketogenic diets really suppress appetite? A systematic review and meta-analysis, *Obes Rev*, 16(1): 64–76.

Gibson, AA, et al., 2017. Strategies to Improve Adherence to Dietary Weight Loss Interventions in Research and Real-World Settings, *Behav Sci*, 7(44): 1–11.

Giovannucci, E, et al., 2010. Diabetes and Cancer: A Consensus Report, *Diabetes Care*, 33: 1674–85.

Goliasch, G, et al., 2015. Premature myocardial infarction is strongly associated with increased levels of remnant cholesterol, *J Clin Lipidol*, 9: 801–6.

Goncalves, MD, et al., 2019. High-fructose corn syrup enhances intestinal tumor growth in mice, Science, 363: 1345–9.

Grabacka, M, et al., 2016. Regulation of Ketone Body Metabolism and the Role of PPARα, *Int J Mol Sci*, 17: 2093.

Gradel, AKJ, et al., 2018. Factors Affecting the Absorption of Subcutaneously Administered Insulin: Effect on Variability, *J Diabetes Res*, 1205121: 17.

Graveling, AJ, et al., 2013. Acute Hypoglycemia Impairs Executive Cognitive Function in Adults With and Without Type 1 Diabetes, *Diabetes Care*, 36: 3240–6.

Gregory, RM, et al., 2017. A Low-Carbohydrate Ketogenic Diet Combined with 6-Weeks of Crossfit Training Improves Body Composition and Performance, *Int J Sports Exerc Med*, 3: 054.

Haahr, H, et al., 2014. A Review of the Pharmacological Properties of Insulin Degludec and Their Clinical Relevance, *Clin Pharmacokinet*, 53: 787–800.

Haffner, SM, 2006. Abdominal obesity, insulin resistance, and cardiovascular risk in pre-diabetes and type 2 diabetes, *Eur Heart J Supp*, 8 (Supplement B): B20–B25.

Hager, SR, et al. 1991. Insulin resistance in normal rats infused with glucose for 72 h, *Am J Physiol Endocrinol Metab*, 260(3): E353–62.

Hall, KD, et al., 2019. Ultra-Processed Diets Cause Excess Calorie Intake and Weight Gain: An Inpatient Randomized Controlled Trial of Ad Libitum Food Intake, *Cell Metab*, 30: 1–11.

Harcombe, Z, et al., 2016. Evidence from randomised controlled trials does not support current dietary fat guidelines: a systematic review and meta-analysis, *Open Heart*, 3: e000409.

Heaney, RP, 2006. Effects of protein on the calcium economy. In: Burckhardt, P, et al., eds. Nutritional aspects of osteoporosis 2006, Lausanne, Switzerland. Amsterdam, Netherlands: Elsevier Inc, 2007: 191–7.

Heaney, RP, et al., 2008. Amount and type of protein influences bone health, *Am J Clin Nutr*, 87(suppl): 1567S–70S.

Heath, GW, et al., 1983. Effects of exercise and lack of exercise on glucose tolerance and insulin sensitivity, *J Appl Physiol*, 55(2): 512–17.

Heinemann, L, et al., 2012. Insulin Infusion Set: The Achilles Heel of Continuous Subcutaneous Insulin Infusion, *J Diabetes Sci Technol*, 6(4): 954–64.

Heinemann, L, et al., 2018. Real-time continuous glucose monitoring in adults with type 1 diabetes and impaired hypoglycaemia awareness or severe hypoglycaemia treated with multiple daily insulin injections (HypoDE): a multicentre, randomised controlled trial, *Lancet*, 391: 1367–77.

Heise, T, et al., 2018. Day-to-Day and Within-Day Variability in Glucose-Lowering Effect Between Insulin Degludec and Insulin Glargine (100 U/mL and 300 U/mL): A Comparison Across Studies, *J Diabetes Sci Technol*, 12(2): 356–63.

Hemkens, LG, et al., 2009. Risk of malignancies in patients with diabetes treated with human insulin or insulin analogues: a cohort study, *Diabetologia*, 52: 1732–44.

Hinshaw, L, et al., 2016. Effect of Pramlintide on Postprandial Glucose Fluxes in Type 1 Diabetes, *J Clin Endocrinol Metab*, 101: 1954–62.

Hirsch, IB, et al., 2005. Should minimal blood glucose variability become the gold standard of glycemic control?, *J Diabetes Complicat*, 19: 178–81.

Hoel, GD, et al., 2016. The risks and benefits of sun exposure 2016, Dermato-Endocrinology, 0(0), e1248325, 17 pages.

Home, PD, et al., 2009. Combined randomised controlled trial experience of malignancies in studies using insulin glargine, *Diabetologia*, 52: 2499–506.

Hu, T, et al., 2016. Effects of a 12-month Low-Carbohydrate Diet vs. a Low-Fat Diet on Bone Mineral Density: A Randomized Controlled Trial, *FASEB J*, 678.12.

Hughes, DS, et al., 2014. Alpha cell function in type 1 diabetes, *Br J Diabetes Vasc Dis*, 14: 45–51.

Hyde, PN, et al., 2019. Dietary carbohydrate restriction improves metabolic syndrome independent of weight loss, *JCI Insight*, 4 (12): e128308.

Institute of Medicine, 2005. Dietary Reference Intakes for Energy, Carbohydrate, Fiber, Fat, Fatty acids, Cholesterol, Protein, and Amino Acids, https://www.nal.usda.gov/sites/default/files/fnic_uploads/energy_full_report.pdf.

Ivanova, EA, et al., 2017. Small Dense Low-Density Lipoprotein as Biomarker for Atherosclerotic Diseases, *Oxid Med Cell Longev*, Article ID 1273042, 1–10.

Jensen, T, et al., 2018. Fructose and Sugar: A Major Mediator of Nonalcoholic Fatty Liver Disease, *J Hepatol*, 68(5): 1063–75.

Johnson, RJ, et al., 2017. Perspective: A Historical and Scientific Perspective of Sugar and Its Relation with Obesity and Diabetes, *Adv Nutr*, 8: 412–22.

Johnson, RJ, et al., 2020. Fructose metabolism as a common evolutionary pathway of survival associated with climate change, food shortage and droughts, *J Intern Med*, 287: 252–62.

Julius, U, et al., 2007. Factors influencing the formation of small dense low-density lipoprotein particles in dependence on the presence of the metabolic syndrome and on the degree of glucose intolerance, *Int J Clin Pract*, 61(11): 1798–1804.

Kaleta, C, et al., 2011. In Silico Evidence for Gluconeogenesis from Fatty Acids in Humans, *PLoS Comput Biol*, 7(7): e1002116.

Kalra, S, 2014. Sodium Glucose Co-Transporter-2 (SGLT2) Inhibitors: A Review of Their Basic and Clinical Pharmacology, *Diabetes Ther*, 5: 355–66.

Karges, B, et al., 2017. Association of Insulin Pump Therapy vs Insulin Injection Therapy With Severe Hypoglycemia, Ketoacidosis, and Glycemic Control Among Children, Adolescents, and Young Adults With Type 1 Diabetes, *JAMA*, 318(14): 1358–66.

Kashiwaya, Y, et al., 1994. Control of Glucose Utilization in Working Perfused Rat Heart, *J Biol Chem*, 269: 25502–14.

Kashiwaya, Y, et al., 1997. Substrate Signaling by Insulin: A Ketone Bodies Ratio Mimics Insulin Action in Heart, *Am J Cardiol*, 80(3): Suppl 1, 50A–64A.

Kessler, SK, et al., 2011. Dietary therapies for epilepsy: Future research, *Epilepsy Behav*, 22(1): 17–22.

Khera, PK, et al., 2008. Evidence for Interindividual Heterogeneity in the Glucose Gradient Across the Human Red Blood Cell Membrane and Its Relationship to Hemoglobin Glycation, *Diabetes*, 57: 2445–52.

Kibirige, D, et al., 2013. Vitamin B12 deficiency among patients with diabetes mellitus: is routine screening and supplementation justified?, *J Diabetes Metab Disord*, 12: 17, 1–6.

King, GL, et al., 2004. Hyperglycemia-induced oxidative stress in diabetic complications, *Histochem Cell Biol*, 122: 333–8.

Kiple, KF, et al., (Editor), 2000. The Cambridge World History of Food (Part 1), Cambridge University Press.

Klonoff, DC, et al., 2018. Investigation of the Accuracy of 18 Marketed Blood Glucose Monitors, *Diabetes Care*, 41(8): 1681–88.

Koeslag, JH, et al., 1980. Post-Exercise Ketosis, *J Physiol*, 301: 79–90.

Koivisto, VA, et al., 1986. Physical Training and Insulin Sensitivity, *Diabetes Metab Rev*, 1(4): 445–81.

Konopka, AR, et al., 2019. Metformin inhibits mitochondrial adaptations to aerobic exercise training in older adults, *Aging Cell*, 18: e12880, 1–12.

Koutnik, AP, et al., 2019. Anticatabolic Effects of Ketone Bodies in Skeletal Muscle, *Trends Endocrinol Metab*, 30(4): 227–9.

Krauss, RM, et al., 2006. Separate effects of reduced carbohydrate intake and weight loss on atherogenic dyslipidemia, *Am J Clin Nutr*, 83: 1025–31.

Kraut, JA, et al., 2010. Metabolic acidosis: pathophysiology, diagnosis and management, *Nat Rev Nephrol*, 6: 274–85.

Krishnasamy, S, et al., 2018. Diabetic Gastroparesis: Principles and Current Trends in Management, *Diabetes Ther*, 9 (Suppl 1): S1–S42.

Kropff, J, et al., 2017. Accuracy and Longevity of an Implantable Continuous Glucose Sensor in the PRECISE Study: A 180-Day, Prospective, Multicenter, Pivotal Trial, *Diabetes Care*, 40: 63–8.

Kuo, PT, et al., 1965. Dietary Sugar in the Production of Hyperglyceridemia, *Ann Int Med*, 62(6): 1199–212.

Lanaspa, MA, et al., 2013. Endogenous fructose production and metabolism in the liver contributes to the development of metabolic syndrome, *Nat Commun*, 4: 2434.

Layman, DK, et al., 2005. Dietary Protein and Exercise Have Additive Effects on Body Composition during Weight Loss in Adult Women, *J Nutr*, 135: 1903–10.

Leal, LG, et al., 2018. Physical Exercise-Induced Myokines and Muscle-Adipose Tissue Crosstalk: A Review of Current Knowledge and the Implications for Health and Metabolic Diseases, *Front Physiol*, 9: 1307.

Lee, JH, et al., 2019. Role of Myokines in Regulating Skeletal Muscle Mass and Function, *Front Physiol*, 10: 42.

Lee, NJ, et al., 2010. Efficacy and Harms of the Hypoglycemic Agent Pramlintide in Diabetes Mellitus, *Ann Fam Med*, 8(6).

Lee, P, et al., 2014. Temperature-Acclimated Brown Adipose Tissue Modulates Insulin Sensitivity in Humans, *Diabetes*, 63: 3686–98.

Lennerz, BS, et al., 2018. Management of type 1 diabetes with a very low-carbohydrate diet, *Pediatrics*, 141(6): 1–10.

Libman, IM, et al., 2003. Changing Prevalence of Overweight Children and Adolescents at Onset of Insulin-Treated Diabetes, *Diabetes Care*, 26: 2871–5.

Liljenquist, JE, et al., 1974. Effects of Glucagon on Lipolysis and Ketogenesis in Normal and Diabetic Men, *J Clin Invest*, 53, 190–7.

Lind, M, et al., 2017. Continuous Glucose Monitoring vs Conventional Therapy for Glycemic Control in Adults With Type 1 Diabetes Treated With Multiple Daily Insulin Injections The GOLD Randomized Clinical Trial, *JAMA*, 317(4): 379–87.

Little, RR, et al., 2009. HbA1c: how do we measure it and what does it mean?, *Curr Opin Endocrinol Diabetes Obes*, 16: 113–8.

Liu-Ambrose, T, et al., 2019. Effect of a Home-Based Exercise Program on Subsequent Falls Among Community-Dwelling High-Risk Older Adults After a Fall A Randomized Clinical Trial, *JAMA*, 321(21): 2092–100.

Liu, C, et al., 2015. Efficacy and Safety of Metformin for Patients with Type 1 Diabetes Mellitus: A Meta-Analysis, *Diabetes Technol Ther*, 17(2).

Liu, LL, et al., 2010. Prevalence of overweight and obesity in youth with diabetes in USA: the SEARCH for Diabetes in Youth Study, *Pediatr Diabetes*, 11(1): 4–11.

Liu, Q, et al., 2014. Vitamin B12 Status in Metformin Treated Patients: Systematic Review, *PLoS ONE*, 9(6): e100379, 1–6.

Liu, Y, et al., 2017. Inflammation: The Common Pathway of Stress-Related Diseases, *Front Hum Neurosci*, 11: 316.

Livingstone, SJ, et al., 2015. Estimated Life Expectancy in a Scottish Cohort With Type 1 Diabetes, 2008-2010, *JAMA*, 313(1): 37–44.

Longland, TM, et al., 2016. Higher compared with lower dietary protein during an energy deficit combined with intense exercise promotes greater lean mass gain and fat mass loss: a randomized trial, *Am J Clin Nutr*, 103: 738–46.

Lu, T, et al. 2019. Pancreatic fat content is associated with β-cell function and insulin resistance in Chinese type 2 diabetes subjects, *Endocr J*, 66(3): 265–70.

Ludwig, DS, 2019. The Ketogenic Diet: Evidence for Optimism but High-Quality Research Needed, *J Nutr*, nxz308.

Ludwig, DS, et al., 2018. The Carbohydrate-Insulin Model of Obesity Beyond "Calories In, Calories Out," *JAMA Intern Med*, 178(8): 1098–103.

Madiraju, AK, et al., 2014. Metformin suppresses gluconeogenesis by inhibiting mitochondrial glycerophosphate dehydrogenase, *Nature*, 510(7506): 542–6.

Maiorino, MI, 2018. The Effects of Subcutaneous Insulin Infusion Versus Multiple Insulin Injections on Glucose Variability in Young Adults with Type 1 Diabetes: The 2-Year Follow-Up of the Observational METRO Study, *Diabetes Technol Ther*, 20(2).

Mäkimattila, S, et al., 2020. Every Fifth Individual With Type 1 Diabetes Suffers From an Additional Autoimmune Disease: A Finnish Nationwide Study, *Diabetes Care*, 43(5): 1041–7.

Malin, SK, et al., 2012. Independent and Combined Effects of Exercise Training and Metformin on Insulin Sensitivity in Individuals With Prediabetes, *Diabetes Care*, 35: 131–6.

Mamerow, MM, et al., 2014. Dietary Protein Distribution Positively Influences 24-h Muscle Protein Synthesis in Healthy Adults, *J Nutr*, 144: 876–80.

Manninen, AH, et al., 2006. Very-low-carbohydrate diets and preservation of muscle mass, *Nutr Metab*, 3(9): 1–4.

Marathe, CS, et al., 2011. Effects of GLP-1 and Incretin-Based Therapies on Gastrointestinal Motor Function, *Exp Diabetes Res*, Article ID 279530, 10 pages.

Mardinoglu, A, et al., 2018. An Integrated Understanding of the Rapid Metabolic Benefits of a Carbohydrate-Restricted Diet on Hepatic Steatosis in Humans, *Cell Metab*, 27: 559–71.

Marliss, EB, et al., 2002. Intense Exercise Has Unique Effects on Both Insulin Release and Its Roles in Glucoregulation: Implications for Diabetes, *Diabetes*, 51 (Suppl. 1): S271–S283.

Martín-Timón, I, et al., 2015. Mechanisms of hypoglycemia unawareness and implications in diabetic patients, *World J Diabetes*, 6(7): 912–26.

Martin, WF, et al., 2005. Dietary protein intake and renal function, *Nutr Metab*, 2(25).

Matsue, M, et al., 2019. Measuring the Antimicrobial Activity of Lauric Acid against Various Bacteria in Human Gut Microbiota Using a New Method, *Cell Transplant*, 28(12): 1528–41.

Mayer-Davis, EJ, et al., 2017. Incidence trends of type 1 and type 2 diabetes among youths, 2002–2012, *N Engl J Med*, 376: 1419–29.

Mazze, RS, et al., 2008. Characterizing glucose exposure for individuals with normal glucose tolerance using continuous glucose monitoring and ambulatory glucose profile analysis, *Diabetes Technol Ther*, 10(3): 149–59.

McCarthy, O, et al., 2019. Resistance Isn't Futile: The Physiological Basis of the Health Effects of Resistance Exercise in Individuals With Type 1 Diabetes, *Front Endocrinol*, 10: 507.

McCarty, MF, et al., 2016. Lauric acid-rich medium-chain triglycerides can substitute for other oils in cooking applications and may have limited pathogenicity, *Open Heart*, 3: e000467.

McEvoy, JW, et al., 2015. Relationship of Cigarette Smoking With Inflammation and Subclinical Vascular Disease, *Arterioscler Thromb Vasc Biol*, 35: 1002–10.

Meirelles, CM, et al., 2016. Effects of Short-Term Carbohydrate Restrictive and Conventional Hypoenergetic Diets and Resistance Training on Strength Gains and Muscle Thickness, *J Sport Sci Med*, 15: 578–84.

Méline, T, 2017. Cold water immersion after exercise: recent data and perspectives on "kaumatherapy," *J Physiol*, 595(9), 2783–4.

Merger, SR, et al., 2016. Prevalence and comorbidities of double diabetes, *Diabetes Res Clin Pr*, 119: 48–56.

Michels, A, et al., 2015. Prediction and Prevention of Type 1 Diabetes: Update on Success of Prediction and Struggles at Prevention, *Pediatr Diabetes*, 16(7): 465–84.

Miller, CT, et al., 2013. The effects of exercise training in addition to energy restriction on functional capacities and body composition in obese adults during weight loss: a systematic review. PLoS One, 8(11): e81692.

Miller, KM, et al., 2015. Current State of Type 1 Diabetes Treatment in the U.S.: Updated Data From the T1D Exchange Clinic Registry, *Diabetes Care*, 38: 971–8.

Miller, VJ, et al., 2018. Nutritional Ketosis and Mitohormesis: Potential Implications for Mitochondrial Function and Human Health, *J Nutr Metab*, Article ID 5157645, 27 pages.

Mitchell, JD, et al., 2018. Impact of Statins on Cardiovascular Outcomes Following Coronary Artery Calcium Scoring, *J Am Coll Cardiol*, 72(25): 3233–42.

Miyashita, Y, et al., 2004, Beneficial effect of low carbohydrate in low calorie diets on visceral fat reduction in type 2 diabetic patients with obesity, *Diabetes Res Clin Pract*, 65, 235–41.

Moore, DR, et al., 2009. Differential stimulation of myofibrillar and sarcoplasmic protein synthesis with protein ingestion at rest and after resistance exercise, *J Physiol*, 587(4): 897–904.

Morrison, DJ, et al., 2016. Formation of short chain fatty acids by the gut microbiota and their impact on human metabolism, *Gut Microbes*, 7(3): 189–200.

Morton, RW, et al., 2018. A systematic review, meta-analysis and meta-regression of the effect of protein supplementation on resistance training-induced gains in muscle mass and strength in healthy adults, *Br J Sports Med*, 52(6): 376–84.

Moser, O, et al., 2016. Accuracy of Continuous Glucose Monitoring (CGM) during Continuous and High-Intensity Interval Exercise in Patients with Type 1 Diabetes Mellitus, *Nutrients*, 8(489): 1–15.

Moss, M, 2013. *Salt Sugar Fat: How the Food Giants Hooked Us*, Penguin Random House Company, New York.

Mottalib, A, et al., 2017. Weight Management in Patients with Type 1 Diabetes and Obesity, *Curr Diab Rep*, 17(10): 92.

Mujica-Parodi, LR, et al., 2020. Diet modulates brain network stability, a biomarker for brain aging, in young adults, *PNAS*, 1913042117.

Müller, WA, et al., 1971. The Effect of Experimental Insulin Deficiency on Glucagon Secretion, *J Clin Invest*, 50: 1992–9.

Mullington, JM, et al., 2010. Sleep Loss and Inflammation, *Best Pract Res Clin Endocrinol Metab*, 24(5): 775–84.

Murphy, CH, et al., 2015. Considerations for protein intake in managing weight loss in athletes, *Eur J Sport Sci*, 15(1): 21–8.

Murray, CJL, et al., 2014. The vast majority of American adults are overweight or obese, and weight is a growing problem among US children, http://www.healthdata.org/news-release/vast-majority-american-adults-are-overweight-or-obese-and-weight-growing-problem-among

Musunuru, K, 2010. Atherogenic Dyslipidemia: Cardiovascular Risk and Dietary Intervention, *Lipids*, 45: 907–14.

Nakagawa, T, et al., 2006. A causal role for uric acid in fructose-induced metabolic syndrome, *Am J Physiol Renal Physiol*, 290: F625–F631.

Nathan, DM, et al, 2008. Translating the A1C Assay Into Estimated Average Glucose Values, *Diabetes Care*, 31: 1–6.

Newman, JC, et al., 2014a. Ketone bodies as signaling metabolites, *Trends Endocrinol Metabol*, 25(1): 42–52.

Newman, JC, et al., 2014b. β-hydroxybutyrate: Much more than a metabolite, *Diabetes Res Clin Pract*, 106(2): 173–81.

Newman, JC, et al., 2017. β-Hydroxybutyrate: A Signaling Metabolite, *Annu Rev Nutr*, 37: 51–76.

Ng, SW, et al., 2012. Use of Caloric and Noncaloric Sweeteners in US Consumer Packaged Foods, 2005-2009, *J Acad Nutr Diet*, 112(11): 1828–34.

Nielsen, JV, et al., 2012. Low carbohydrate diet in type 1 diabetes, long-term improvement and adherence: A clinical audit, *Diabetol Metab Syndr*, 4: 23.

Nyenwe, EA, et al., 2016. The evolution of diabetic ketoacidosis: An update of its etiology, pathogenesis and management, *Metabolism*, 65: 507–21.

Ormazabal, V, et al., 2018. Association between insulin resistance and the development of cardiovascular disease, *Cardiovasc Diabetol*, 17: 122.

Osler, SW, 1920. *The Principles and Practice of Medicine: Designed for the Use of Practitioners and Students of Medicine*, page 433, https://ia802608.us.archive.org/3/items/principlesandpr00mccrgoog/principlesandpr00mccrgoog.pdf.

Osna, NA, 2010. Alcohol, inflammation, and gut-liver-brain interactions in tissue damage and disease development, *World J Gastroenterol*, 16(11): 1304–13.

Owen, OE, 2005. Ketone Bodies as a Fuel for the Brain during Starvation, *Biochem Mol Biol Edu*, 33(4): 246–51.

Owen, OE, et al., 1967. Brain Metabolism during Fasting, *J Clin Invest*, 46(10): 1589–95.

Owens, DR, 2012. Glargine and Cancer: Can We Now Suggest Closure?, *Diabetes Care*, 35: 2426–28.

Paddon-Jones, D, et al., 2008. Protein, weight management, and satiety, *Am J Clin Nutr*, 87 (suppl): 1558S–61S.

Paddon-Jones, D, et al., 2010. Dietary protein recommendations and the prevention of sarcopenia: Protein, amino acid metabolism and therapy, *Curr Opin Clin Nutr Metab Care*, Jan. 1: 1–9.

Palgi A, et al., 1985. Multidisciplinary Treatment of Obesity with a Protein-sparing Modified Fast: Results in 668 Outpatients, *Am J Public Health*, 75: 1190–4.

Paoli, A, et al., 2012. Ketogenic diet does not affect strength performance in elite artistic gymnasts, *J Int Soc Sports Nutr*, 9: 34.

Paoli, A, et al., 2013. Beyond weight loss: a review of the therapeutic uses of very-low-carbohydrate (ketogenic) diets, *Eur J Clin Nutr*, 67: 789–96.

Parsons, TJ, et al., 2017. Physical Activity, Sedentary Behavior, and Inflammatory and Hemostatic Markers in Men, *Med Sci Sports Exerc*, 49(3): 459–65.

Patterson, E, et al., 2012. Health Implications of High Dietary Omega-6 Polyunsaturated Fatty Acids, *J Nutr Metab*, Article ID 539426, 16 pages.

Peters, AL, et al., 2015. Euglycemic Diabetic Ketoacidosis: A Potential Complication of Treatment With Sodium–Glucose Cotransporter 2 Inhibition, *Diabetes Care*, 38: 1687–93.

Pettus, J, et al., 2018. Recommendations for Initiating Use of Afrezza Inhaled Insulin in Individuals with Type 1 Diabetes, *Diabetes Technol Ther*, 20(6): 448–51.

Phillips, SM, 2014. A Brief Review of Higher Dietary Protein Diets in Weight Loss: A Focus on Athletes, *Sports Med*, 44 (Suppl 2): S149–S153.

Polonsky, KS, et al., 1988. Quantitative Study of Insulin Secretion and Clearance in Normal and Obese Subjects, *J Clin Invest*, 81: 435–41.

Porcellati, F, et al., 2013. Thirty Years of Research on the Dawn Phenomenon: Lessons to Optimize Blood Glucose Control in Diabetes, *Diabetes Care*, 36: 3860–2.

Porte, Jr, R, et al., 1997. *Ellenberg & Rifkin's Diabetes Mellitus*, 5th edition, Appleton & Lange.

Price, WA, 1939. *Nutrition and Physical Degeneration* published by the Price-Pottenger Nutrition Foundation, 20th printing, 2011.

Priya, G, et al., 2018. A Review of Insulin Resistance in Type 1 Diabetes: Is There a Place for Adjunctive Metformin?, *Diabetes Ther*, 9: 349–61.

Ramsden, CE, et al., 2010. n-6 Fatty acid-specific and mixed polyunsaturate dietary interventions have different effects on CHD risk: a meta-analysis of randomised controlled trials, *Br J Nutr*, 104: 1586–600.

Ravnskov, U, et al., 2014. The Questionable Benefits of Exchanging Saturated Fat With Polyunsaturated Fat, *Mayo Clin Proc*, 89(4): 451–3.

Reaven, GM, et al., 1967. Role of Insulin in Endogenous Hypertriglyceridemia, *J Clin Invest*, 46(11): 1756–67.

Reed, BG, et al., 2018. The Normal Menstrual Cycle and the Control of Ovulation. https://www.ncbi.nlm.nih.gov/books/NBK279054/

Regnell, SE, et al., 2011. Hepatic Steatosis in Type 1 Diabetes, *Rev Diabetes Stud*, 8: 454–67.

Reinke, H, et al., 2019. Crosstalk between metabolism and circadian clocks, *Nature Reviews Molecular Cell Biology*, 20: 227–41.

Reiterer, F, et al., 2017. Significance and Reliability of MARD for the Accuracy of CGM Systems, *J Diabetes Sci Technol*, 11(1): 59–67.

Reno, CM, et al., 2013. Severe Hypoglycemia–Induced Lethal Cardiac Arrhythmias Are Mediated by Sympathoadrenal Activation, *Diabetes*, 62: 3570–81.

Rewers, M, et al., 2018. The Environmental Determinants of Diabetes in the Young (TEDDY) Study: 2018 Update, *Curr Diab Rep*, 18(136): 1–14.

Riddle, MC, et al., 2020. Standards of Medical Care in Diabetes – 2020, *Diabetes Care*, 43, Suppl. 1: S1–S212.

Roberts, CK, et al., 2013. Metabolic Syndrome and Insulin Resistance: Underlying Causes and Modification by Exercise Training, *Compr Physiol*, 3: 1–58.

Rohlfing, CL, et al., 2002. Defining the relationship between plasma glucose and HbA1c: analysis of glucose profiles and HbA1c in the Diabetes Control and Complications Trial, *Diabetes Care*, 25: 275–8.

Rosenstock, J, et al., 2009. Similar risk of malignancy with insulin glargine and neutral protamine Hagedorn (NPH) insulin in patients with type 2 diabetes: findings from a 5 year randomised, open-label study, *Diabetologia*, 52: 1971–3.

Rosenstock, J, et al., 2015, Euglycemic Diabetic Ketoacidosis: A Predictable, Detectable, and Preventable Safety Concern With SGLT2 Inhibitors, *Diabetes Care*, 38: 1638–42.

Runyan, KR, 2019. What you need to know about a low-carb diet and your kidneys, https://www.dietdoctor.com/low-carb/kidney-health

Rzepka-Migut, B, et al., 2020. Melatonin-Measurement Methods and the Factors Modifying the Results. A Systematic Review of the Literature, *Int J Environ Res Public Health*, 17(1916): 1–18.

Saad, A, et al., 2012. Diurnal Pattern to Insulin Secretion and Insulin Action in Healthy Individuals, *Diabetes*, 61(11): 2691–700.

Sävendahl, L, et al., 1999. Fasting Increases Serum Total Cholesterol, LDL Cholesterol and Apolipoprotein B in Healthy, Nonobese Humans, *J Nutr*, 129(11): 2005–8.

Secrest, AM, et al., 2011. Characterising sudden death and dead-in-bed syndrome in Type 1 diabetes: Analysis from 2 childhood-onset Type 1 diabetes registries, *Diabet Med*, 28(3): 293–300.

Selvin, E, et al., 2014. Fructosamine and glycated albumin for risk stratification and prediction of incident diabetes and microvascular complications: a prospective cohort analysis of the Atherosclerosis Risk in Communities (ARIC) study, *Lancet Diabetes Endocrinol*, 2(4): 279–88.

Semenkovich, CF, 2006. Insulin Resistance and Atherosclerosis, *J Clin Invest*, 116: 1813–22.

Shaffer, PA, 1921. Antiketogenesis. II. The Ketogenic Antiketogenic Balance In Man, *J Biol Chem*, 47: 449–73.

Sheikh-Ali, M, et al., 2008. Can Serum β-Hydroxybutyrate Be Used to Diagnose Diabetic Ketoacidosis?, *Diabetes Care*, 31(4): 643–7.

Shimazu, T, et al., 2013. Suppression of Oxidative Stress by β-Hydroxybutyrate, an Endogenous Histone Deacetylase Inhibitor, *Science*, 339(6116): 211–4.

Simpson, SJ, et al., 2005. Obesity: the protein leverage hypothesis, *Obesity Reviews*, 6: 133–42.

Skrivarhaug, T, et al., 2006. Long-term mortality in a nationwide cohort of childhood-onset type 1 diabetic patients in Norway, *Diabetologia*, 49: 298–305.

Snieder, H, et al., 2001. HbA1c Levels Are Genetically Determined Even in Type 1 Diabetes Evidence From Healthy and Diabetic Twins, *Diabetes*, 50: 2858–63.

Soupal, J, et al., 2014. Glycemic variability is higher in type 1 diabetes patients with microvascular complications irrespective of glycemic control, *Diabetes Technol Ther*, 16(4).

St-Pierre, AC, et al., 2005. Low-Density Lipoprotein Subfractions and the Long-Term Risk of Ischemic Heart Disease in Men, *Arterioscler Thromb Vasc Biol*, 25: 553–9.

Steinberg, D, et al., 1971. Principles of Nutrition and Dietary Recommendations for Patients with Diabetes Mellitus, *Diabetes*, 20(9): 633–4.

Stenström, G, et al., 2005. Latent Autoimmune Diabetes in Adults, *Diabetes*, 54 (Suppl. 2): S68–S72.

Swift, DL, et al., 2014. The Role of Exercise and Physical Activity in Weight Loss and Maintenance, *Prog Cardiovasc Dis*, 56(4): 441–7.

Taleb, N, et al., 2016. Comparison of Two Continuous Glucose Monitoring Systems, Dexcom G4 Platinum and Medtronic Paradigm Veo Enlite System, at Rest and During Exercise, *Diabetes Technol Ther*, 18(9): 561–7.

Taubes, G, 2007. *Good Calories, Bad Calories: Fats, Carbs, and the Controversial Science of Diet and Health*, Alfred A. Knopf, New York.

Taubes, G, 2016. *The Case Against Sugar*, Alfred A. Knopf, New York.

Tauschmann, M, et al., 2018. Closed-loop insulin delivery in suboptimally controlled type 1 diabetes: a multicentre, 12-week randomised trial, *Lancet*, 392: 1321–9.

Teicholz, N, 2010. *The Big Fat Surprise: Why Butter, Meat and Cheese Belong in a Healthy Diet*, Simon & Schuster, New York.

Thaker, VV, 2017. Genetic And Epigenetic Causes Of Obesity, *Adolesc Med State Art Rev*, 28(2): 379–405.

The 2015–2020 Dietary Guidelines for Americans https://health.gov/dietaryguidelines/2015/

The DCCT Research Group, 1993a. Nutrition interventions for intensive therapy in the Diabetes Control and Complications Trial, *J Am Diet Assoc*, 93: 768–72.

The DCCT Research Group, 1993b. The Effect of Intensive Treatment of Diabetes on the Development and Progression of Long-Term Complications in Insulin-Dependent Diabetes Mellitus, *N Engl J Med*, 329: 977–86.

The DCCT/EDIC Study Research Group, 2005. Intensive Diabetes Treatment and Cardiovascular Disease in Patients with Type 1 Diabetes, *N Engl J Med*, 353(25): 2643–53.

Thomas, D, et al., 2009. Low glycaemic index, or low glycaemic load, diets for diabetes mellitus, *Cochrane Database Syst Rev*, Issue 1. Art. No.: CD006296.

Thomas, F, et al., 2016. Blood Glucose Levels of Subelite Athletes During 6 Days of Free Living, *J Diabetes Sci Technol*, 10(6): 1335–43.

Thomas, NJ, et al., 2018. Frequency and phenotype of type 1 diabetes in the first six decades of life: a cross-sectional, genetically stratified survival analysis from UK Biobank, *Lancet Diabetes Endocrinol*, 6(2): 122–9.

Thongtang, N, et al., 2017. Metabolism and proteomics of large and small dense LDL in combined hyperlipidemia: effects of rosuvastatin, *J Lipid Res*, 58: 1315–24.

Thorpe, MP, et al., 2008. A diet high in protein, dairy, and calcium attenuates bone loss over twelve months of weight loss and maintenance relative to a conventional high-carbohydrate diet in adults, *J Nutr*, 138: 1096–100.

Ting, RZ, et al., 2006. Risk Factors of Vitamin B12 Deficiency in Patients Receiving Metformin, *Arch Intern Med*, 166(18): 1975–9.

Tsai, MY, et al., 2014. New Automated Assay of Small Dense Low-Density Lipoprotein Cholesterol Identifies Risk of Coronary Heart Disease, *Arterioscler Thromb Vasc Biol*, 34: 196–201.

Uchida, K, 2003. 4-Hydroxy-2-nonenal: a product and mediator of oxidative stress, *Prog Lipid Res*, 42: 318–43.

Umpierrez, GE, et al., 2019. Diabetic Ketoacidosis and Hyperglycemic Hyperosmolar Syndrome, *JAMA*, 321(11).

Unger, RH, et al., 2012. Glucagonocentric restructuring of diabetes: a pathophysiologic and therapeutic makeover, *J Clin Invest*, 122(1): 4–12.

Van Belle, TL, et al., 2011. Type 1 Diabetes: Etiology, Immunology, and Therapeutic Strategies, *Physiol Rev*, 91: 79–118.

VanderWeele JJ, et al., 2014. Antecedent recurrent hypoglycemia reduces lethal cardiac arrhythmias induced by severe hypoglycemia in diabetic rats, *Diabetes*, 53 (Suppl. 1): A39.

Vasudevan, S, et al., 2014. Interference of Intravenous Vitamin C With Blood Glucose Testing, *Diabetes Care*, 37: e93–e94.

Veech, RL, et al., 2001. Ketone Bodies, Potential Therapeutic Uses, *IUBMB Life*, 51: 241–7.

Viana, RB, et al., 2019. Is interval training the magic bullet for fat loss? A systematic review and meta-analysis comparing moderate-intensity continuous training with high-intensity interval training (HIIT), *Br J Sports Med*, 53: 655–64.

Volek, JS, et al., 2002. Body Composition and Hormonal Responses to a Carbohydrate-Restricted Diet, *Metabolism*, 51(7): 864–70.

Volek, JS, et al., 2005. Modification of Lipoproteins by Very Low-Carbohydrate Diets, *J Nutr*, 135: 1339–42.

Volek, JS, et al., 2008. Dietary carbohydrate restriction induces a unique metabolic state positively affecting atherogenic dyslipidemia, fatty acid partitioning, and metabolic syndrome, *Prog Lipid Res*, 47(5): 307–18.

Volek, JS, et al., 2011a. The Art and Science of Low Carbohydrate Living, Beyond Obesity, LLC.

Volek, JS, et al., 2011b. The Art and Science of Low Carbohydrate Performance, Beyond Obesity, LLC.

Volek, JS, et al., 2016. Metabolic characteristics of keto-adapted ultra-endurance runners, *Metabolism*, 65(3): 100–10.

Volk, BM, et al., 2014. Effects of Step-Wise Increases in Dietary Carbohydrate on Circulating Saturated Fatty Acids and Palmitoleic Acid in Adults with Metabolic Syndrome, *PLoS ONE*, 9(11): e113605.

Volkow, ND, et al., 2011. Reward, dopamine and the control of food intake: implications for obesity, *Trends Cogn Sci*, 15(1): 37–46.

Wall, BT, et al., 2015. Aging Is Accompanied by a Blunted Muscle Protein Synthetic Response to Protein Ingestion, *PLoS One*, 10(11): e0140903.

Walton, RG, et al., 2019. Metformin blunts muscle hypertrophy in response to progressive resistance exercise training in older adults: A randomized, double-blind, placebo-controlled, multicenter trial: The MASTERS trial, *Aging Cell*, 00: e13039, 1–19.

Wang, H, et al., 2019. Skeletal Muscle Mass as a Mortality Predictor among Nonagenarians and Centenarians: A Prospective Cohort Study, *Scientific Reports*, 9: 2420.

Washburn, RA, et al. 2014. Does the method of weight loss effect long-term changes in weight, body composition or chronic disease risk factors in overweight or obese adults? A systematic review. PLoS One, 9(10): e109849.

What Americans Eat, 2010. Top 10 sources of calories in the U.S. diet, https://www.health.harvard.edu/healthy-eating/top-10-sources-of-calories-in-the-us-diet

Wilson, GJ, et al., 2012. Post-Meal Responses of Elongation Factor 2 (eEF2) and Adenosine Monophosphate-Activated Protein Kinase (AMPK) to Leucine and Carbohydrate Supplements for Regulating Protein Synthesis Duration and Energy Homeostasis in Rat Skeletal Muscle, *Nutrients*, 4(11): 1723–39.

Withrow, CD, 1980. The ketogenic diet: mechanism of anticonvulsant action. *Adv Neurol*, 7: 635–42.

Wolever, TMS, et al., 1991. The glycemic index: methodology and clinical implications. *Am J Clin Nutr*, 54: 846–54.

Wolfsdorf, JI, et al., 2019. SGLT Inhibitors for Type 1 Diabetes: Proceed With Extreme Caution, *Diabetes Care*, 42: 991–3.

Wolfson, JA, et al., 2015. Is cooking at home associated with better diet quality or weight-loss intention? *Public Health Nutr*, 18(8): 1397–406.

World Health Organization Says Processed Meat Causes Cancer, https://www.cancer.org/latest-news/world-health-organization-says-processed-meat-causes-cancer.html

Wu, JW, et al., 2014. Commonly used diabetes and cardiovascular medications and cancer recurrence and cancer-specific mortality: a review of the literature, *Expert Opin Drug Saf*, 13(8): 1071–99.

Yang, H, et al., 2018. Lauric Acid Is an Inhibitor of Clostridium difficile Growth in Vitro and Reduces Inflammation in a Mouse Infection Model, *Front Microbiol*, 8: 2635.

Yang, Q, 2010. Gain weight by "going diet?" Artificial sweeteners and the neurobiology of sugar cravings, *Yale J Biol Med*, 83: 101–8.

Yardley, JE, et al., 2012. Effects of Performing Resistance Exercise Before Versus After Aerobic Exercise on Glycemia in Type 1 Diabetes, *Diabetes Care*, 35: 669–75.

Yardley, JE, et al., 2013. Resistance Versus Aerobic Exercise: Acute effects on glycemia in type 1 diabetes, *Diabetes Care*, 36: 537–42.

Yasuda, J, et al., 2020. Evenly Distributed Protein Intake over 3 Meals Augments Resistance Exercise–Induced Muscle Hypertrophy in Healthy Young Men, *J Nutr*, 00: 1–7.

Yeung, EH, et al., 2010. Longitudinal Study of Insulin Resistance and Sex Hormones over the Menstrual Cycle: The BioCycle Study, *J Clin Endocrinol Metab*, 95: 5435–42.

Youm, Y, et al., 2015. Ketone body β-hydroxybutyrate blocks the NLRP3 inflammasome-mediated inflammatory disease, *Nat Med*, 21(3): 263–9.

Zhang, T, et al., 2018. Beneficial Effect of Intestinal Fermentation of Natural Polysaccharides, *Nutrients*, 10: 1055.

Zhang, Y, et al., 2013. Ketosis proportionately spares glucose utilization in brain, *J Cereb Blood Flow Metab*, 33: 1307–11.

Zheng, P, et al., 2018. Gut microbiome in type 1 diabetes: A comprehensive review, *Diabetes Metab Res Rev*, 34: e3043, 1–9.

Zhou, J, et al., 2009. Reference values for continuous glucose monitoring in Chinese subjects, *Diabetes Care*, 32: 1188–93.

Zhou, J, et al., 2011. Establishment of normal reference ranges for glycemic variability in Chinese subjects using continuous glucose monitoring, *Med Sci Monit*, 17(1): CR9–13.

Zilberter, T, et al., 2018. Ketogenic Ratio Determines Metabolic Effects of Macronutrients and Prevents Interpretive Bias, *Front Nutr*, 5: 75.

CPSIA information can be obtained
at www.ICGtesting.com
Printed in the USA
LVHW092014141220
674149LV00030BA/432